The Trap of Proximity Violence

Ignazia Bartholini

The Trap of Proximity Violence

Research and Insights into Male Dominance and Female Resistance

Springer

Ignazia Bartholini
University of Palermo
Palermo, Italy

ISBN 978-3-030-52450-0 ISBN 978-3-030-52451-7 (eBook)
https://doi.org/10.1007/978-3-030-52451-7

This Springer imprint is published by the registered company Springer Nature Switzerland AG
The registered company address is: Gewerbestrasse 11, 6330 Cham, Switzerland

Preface

The links between violence against women/gender-based violence and patriarchy have been explored at length by contemporary sociological literature. They describe an order of things firmly rooted in societies. They are rooted in the Western world even when it comes to the illusory crisis of this ominous binomial; they are rooted in the rest of the world where the same effects are clearly visible. Less travelled, though not completely unexplored, is the pathway that highlights the links between vulnerability and proximity violence, meant as a synthesis which reaches beyond patriarchal/post-patriarchal polarisation. Unknown is also the *topos* of convergence between resistance and regressive mestizament, which today defines one of the main constitutive junctions of its perpetuation. The violence trap lies precisely at the intersection between resistance against acknowledgement of violence by victims and nostalgia for an order of relationships once the basis of a social system felt by women who are not direct victims of that same violence.

The investigative aim of this book is to bring to light the crevasses where violence lurks ready to return in disguise as well as the lairs where it hides. Like a whirlwind, violence appears in all its destructive might and disappears. Precisely because violence is of a proxemic kind, it is hard to position with respect to those who wish to objectify it. Its screens are many and the causes that feed it are endowed with a good dose of relational and lexical ambiguity. Because it is profoundly unjust, unfair, wrong and at the same time intimate and socio-emotional, it is often justifiable and justified by victims themselves.

It is a matter of having procedural violence assert itself where structural violence has failed. By structural violence, we mean an entire system of values which sustains and backs the removal of the feminine, by objectifying and reifying bodies, while male and heterosexual desire is the measure by which public life and social spaces are defined. By procedural violence is meant the attempt to establish a gender regime where it has lost part of its normative strength. Proximity violence is more ambiguous and elusive, but it permeates relationships along both the vertical axis of social stratifications and the horizontal axis of different cultures.

Using specific disciplinary terminology, this violence is considered "close-at-hand violence" and is used to underline the way in which it is perpetrated by the "closest person in the relationship of reference". This kind of violence is (1) self-sufficient, (2) auto-immune and (3) conflict-excluding (Bartholini, 2019). It lies within the oppressive, ritual context constituting the keystone of the relationship and defines the reciprocal identities of the participants during violent interaction, in the variety of modes it uses to manifest itself, i.e. physical, psychological and symbolic. A close-at-hand type of violence can only be implemented if it is ritual, like the staging of a show; it envisages both direct (offspring and relatives) and indirect (friends, neighbours and work colleagues) onlookers. These assume a crucial function in the actual staging of the violent performance, consenting the subjects involved in the drama to assume roles and identities they lack in actual public life. Ignazia Bartholini examines some of the main theoretical aspects of the contemporary debate regarding violence and close relationships, and compares them through the lives and experiences of Sicilian women.

This common scenario underlines how concepts of power and domination – especially those of immigrant cultures – practices of objectification, commodification and female exploitation, reach a peak which, in extreme cases becomes manipulation, even annihilation of the victim. Violence from this angle is an oppressive behavioural practice used to control the weakest to the full advantage of the strongest – a phenomenon increased by devastating effects it has on women. Every act, every gesture, every violent ritual has its own specific traits regarding the relationship, the context and the institutions; but violence, as a category, contains "matryoshka-like" interpretative dimensions involving different levels that refract, mix and mingle.

If we divide violence according to its perspective planes, we multiply types of gender-based violence to measure each on the basis of social and statistical indicators. A similar operation does not produce a critical consideration of the empirical and symbolic structures that arise within gender relations between women and men and, intersectionally speaking, between women who perceive or deny the violence their sisters and cousins experience, while in Mediterranean Europe the post-patriarchal structure of gender relations is far from being questioned in terms of stereotypes and behavioural practices.

In other words, we are used to thinking of violence as something that belongs to the "other" cultures of men and women from "other" continents, to "other" collective histories and to the lack of development of "others", as if a phenomenology of the spirit still needed to be accomplished elsewhere while the *Weltgeist* is embodied primarily in the advanced West.

We also imagine that violence belongs to the culture of slums and acts as a glue in the crevasses of European society attributable to the borderlines of marginality, to material and social poverty, a stratification that goes hand in hand with the crystallisation of male domination.

This volume seeks, therefore, to cross all these planes: emigration and migrant cultures still closed like chrysalises in misogynous worlds based on the possession of the female body (Chap. 2), the physical exploitation of the body of European women from poorer countries by men who live in other European countries (Chap. 3), cultural plane of a Mediterranean Europe which still preserves an intrinsically segregationist culture (Chap. 4) and, finally, the more subtle and underground plane of nostalgia for a reassuring violent system (Chap. 5).

We would like to imagine this volume as the perimeter of a polyhedron where the surfaces correspond to the different scenarios of the violence which connotes the segregation of sub-Saharan women, the sexual exploitation of Romanian women and, again, the faltering violence of women from the popular districts of Palermo. This means carrying out an operation of disenchantment regarding the now classical vision of violence, which does regard gender, is against women and can be analysed upon several levels. This is also a form of violence that victims legitimise and justify to some extent within the relationships which deplete their bodies and identities while, at the same time, triggering mechanisms of emotional resistance. It is, as I shall try to explain here, a particular form of violence that the author indicates as "proximal". Violence acts only within relationships supported by an emotional exchange, warm emotions, feelings that convey the need to receive comfort, complicity and support. This is a type of violence that when not experienced becomes nostalgia for a forsaken identity; this is a covert form of violence which feeds on female vulnerability and triggers practices of resistance which jeopardise objective evaluation.

In the public sphere, economic reasons direct the rules of profit and favour the elimination of emotions. It is a *Zweckrationalität* (Weber, 1922) which obliges the forces that direct its utilitarian functions to appear as a "civilisation of instinct" also at a cultural level. In the private sphere, violence – experienced or witnessed – is a reflexive response to a need for emotions that have been eliminated from the public and professional sphere. This volume aims at highlighting with extreme clarity the self and the hetero-referential traps that proximity violence and its dynamics generate, thanks to the interpretations they are given at the institutional level (Chap. 3), at linguistic performativity (Chap, 4) and at a certain type of opinion defined according to gender difference (Chap. 5).

Chapter 1 develops an argumentative plot to identify the elements which denote proximity violence as a kind of violence, which transcends the concepts of "violence against women" and "gender-based violence" and which finds fertile terrain in the vulnerability of women involved in migration.

Chapter 2, referring to the gender-violence binomial, highlights some of the dynamics between "resistant victims" and "close-at-hand perpetrators", which characterise proximity violence. The roles played within gender dynamics among migrants are used to throw light on possible processes by which mechanisms of submission to and normalisation of gender violence seem to be internalised by these victims of proximity violence, emphasising the viscous links existing between vulnerability and resistance. It also seeks to highlight equivocations surrounding affective action declined in feminine terms and instrumental action in masculine terms, suggesting that proximity may be considered a more "intimate and deceptive" declension of gender violence.

Chapter 3 delves into legal interpretations of trafficking – a macroscopic phenomenon of tragic violence because it is thus shifted to the level of commodification, a symbolic exchange between identity and sex and the material exchange of body and money, acknowledged as a category of vulnerability. It analyses the concept of vulnerability as related to proximity violence, which evolves, in a specific way, into "proximal vulnerability", as a "means" used by the trafficker and clarified through some of the rulings of the Italian and Romanian courts.

Chapter 4 emphasises the ongoing character of a late modernity still hanging in the balance between frameworks of representation and legitimisation of woman and roles she plays in the public sphere by virtue of the emancipation that has taken place and the contradictions which emerge due to attempts to reconcile old and new models of femininity. The chapter also explores the effects of the proximity violence experienced by migrant women on how they and the issue are perceived by the autochthonous women living in the *Ballarò* district. It highlights the signs of regressive mestizament that surface, the effects of which are testified by the reflections of the native Palermitan women who assess the behaviour of the immigrant women positively, due to their respect for traditional moral mores and everyday lives which in those social circles are characterised by gender and family segregation.

Chapter 5 describes the modes and verbal ploys used (in the various public and private contexts where they conduct their relationships) to communicate the effects of symbolic violence that describe how genders play their respective identitarian roles. It underlines the semantic significance of the language of violence rooted in Mediterranean culture. To this end, the author refers to "euphemised discourse" (Bourdieu, 1982) and the concept of "agency" (Duranti, 2007) used to describe the process of naturalisation of discursive practices geared towards affirming the androcentric system of language. Against this background, the legacy of a Mediterranean culture, which remains patriarchal and sexist, was examined through discourse analysis of several stories by Andrea Camilleri and the foregrounding of certain "gender-oriented" dialectal lexemes. Violence as "proximal violence" is not described in terms merely of its procedural effect, but is analysed with regard to its cultural aspects, rooted in the shame-and-honour paradigm of the Mediterranean area and compared to the epochal crisis of masculine identity.

Finally, Chap. 6 focuses on the unfinished nature of a kind of late modernity hovering on the cusp between frameworks of representation and legitimisation of woman and the roles she plays publicly because of the emancipation that has taken place while examining the contradictions which emerge when efforts are made to reconcile old and new models of femininity. We shall try, therefore, to loosen some of the knots regarding relationships between gender violence and "cultural representations". We shall focus, above all, on the "adaptive preferences" and "corrosive disadvantages" that mingle in the private lives of European women, in total contrast with their social advances, and favoured by conditions of emotional oppression and that very habitus where the ups and downs of the past are immanent in a hybrid present of which contemporary women are often the unknowing amphibiotic bearers. It is a matter of excess images whose charms and horrors lie in the disturbing juxtaposition of two opposite registers. In these we can see the ups and downs of the existence of many women, their aspirations to greatness, their sense of helplessness and fears of the unknown (Augé, 2000). Each of the women interviewed who was known to us and who contributed to the creation of this volume, is an extended and situated self which, in its freedom or non-freedom of action, encompasses a principle of authority (membership of a community or family, belonging to a tradition, a culture) equally essential to the definition of resistant aspects of her as a person.

References

Augé, M. (2000). *Fictions fin de siècle suivi de Que se passe-t-il?*. Paris, France: Librairie Arthème Fayard.
Bartholini, I. (2019). *Proximity violence in migration times. A focus in some regions of Italy, France, Spain*. Milano, Italy: FrancoAngeli.
Bourdieu, P. (1982). *Se que parler veut dir. L'économie des echanges linguistiques*. Paris, France: Fayard
Duranti, A. (2007). *Etnopragmatica. La forza nel parlare*. Rome, Italy: Carocci Editore
Weber, M. (1922). *Wirtschaft und Gesellschaft*. Tübingen, Germany: Mohr

Contents

Chapter 1
Violence and Proximity Violence: Links and Interpretative Developments

1.1 Introduction

Recent female migration flows undergo rethinking when addressed by discussion regarding gender relations, since these concern the social and cultural significance of the female bodies, of their exposure to the *vulnus* of violence within the context of contemporary migration. The exposition of women to risk becomes chronic when institutions are unable to guarantee the fundamental rights of human beings, like bodily health and integrity, personal dignity, and safeguard against any kind of violence (Nussbaum, 2011). The extreme variety of migrant women's experiences is reflected in the diversity of the situations where they undergo discrimination and maltreatment. Gender relations in areas of the Mediterranean cannot be interpreted by applying any single currently shared paradigm but are themselves the product of a hybrid cluster of diverse cultural influences, which nevertheless reconstitute a puzzle, one constituting a bridge between the different shores of the Mediterranean (Bartholini, 2015; Butler, 2011; Corradi, 2005; Wiederman, 2000).

Just as there is an Atlantic Europe, there is also a Mediterranean one, which borders on the Muslim world, in its Arabic, Persian, Kurdish, Turkish variants, as well as on the East. A geographic dimension is, above all, a cultural one, despite Edward Said (1993) having claimed that the Mediterranean was merely an invention of the West. The Mediterranean is, today, a crucible of cultural models – some old, some new – where some behavioural patterns, based on gender violence, are legitimated by centuries-old sexist logic and patriarchal reverberations. They intertwine according to the principle known as "intercommunicating vessels" and reinforce those elements which, through residual in Mediterranean Europe, manage to strengthen a Mediterranean culture in its anachronistic elements and in the danger of its effects. The Mediterranean culture stands on the margins of the "philo-Atlantic assemblages" without interfering with its pre-established hierarchies (Cassano & Zolo, 2007). There exists, actually, a culturally dominant West and many other subordinate "Western souths" whose scarce cultural (and economic) relevance permits the

I. Bartholini, *The Trap of Proximity Violence*,
https://doi.org/10.1007/978-3-030-52451-7_1

persistence of contexts of life where the law of the fittest applies, and like in the jungle, the vulnerability of the weakest exposes them to constant risks of violence.

In southern Europe, the most recent migratory arrivals have also contributed to the re-emergence of the "honour-and-shame" paradigm (Appiah, 2010; Giordano, 1994; Mackenzie, Rogers, & Dodds, 2014), expressed primarily through gender-oriented relations founded on control of women within marital and parental relationships. As Bimbi (2015) wrote recently, the honour-and-shame paradigm is a characteristic of the Mediterranean area. Although it seems to represent an archaic residue, it continues to spread through the groups of newcomers, also in terms of blatant violence.

One of the most devastating effects of this paradigm is legitimization of the sexual exploitation of migrants mainly from the African continent (especially Nigeria) but from Eastern Europe too (especially Romania). Furthermore, it emphasizes forms of gender submission found within more traditional marriage-based relationships. The issue of female subordination and exploitation may, therefore, be attributed to the cultural models underlying the socialization processes experienced by migrant women in their native countries and reproduced in their host countries. Female subordination does not belong to "them" or to "us" but creates a link between the countries of origin and destination when it comes to the reproduction of male domination (Bourdieu, 1998). The logical, consequential assumption is that there is almost always a continuum between situations of domination and exploitation and the perpetration of violent acts against women (Collins, 2008; Filosof, 2000; Gillioz, De Puy, & Ducret, 2000; Råheim et al. 2016; Razack et al., 2011).

The consideration of violence as an expression of the "normality" of relationships characterized by female submission and, in extreme cases, by sexual exploitation proves sociologically useful to in-depth studies of processes and representations which contribute to the perpetuation of male power within gender relations in some migratory contexts. The more representations legitimizing the centuries-old exercise of control by men over women's bodies are shared socially, the more they relegate women to positions of subjugation and segregation.

In this chapter the author analyses some of the role positions emerging from the gender dynamics found among migrants. She aims at shedding light on possible processes of submission and internalization of mechanisms of gender subalternity of migrants and on the viscous links between vulnerability (Fineman, 2008) and resilience (Bracke, 2016). She also proposes highlighting equivocations surrounding affective action declined in feminine terms and instrumental action declined in masculine terms, suggesting that proximity may be considered a more "intimate and deceptive" declension of gender violence. Women degrade their bodies through sexual exploitation (and not just that), if accompanied by positive feelings towards the perpetrator (affective action). In the perpetrator, the positive feelings belong most of the time to a strategy aimed at exploiting the victim's body (instrumental action). The affective action of the one and the instrumental action of the other, however, have remote cultural roots, stemming from a complex mixture of power, prejudice, and patriarchalism.

1.2 Domination Over and Segregation of the Female Body

The concept of patriarchy is indispensable, therefore, when attempting to analyse gender inequality: "the concept and theory of patriarchy is essential to capture the depth, pervasiveness and interconnectedness of different aspects of women's subordination, and can be developed in such a way as to take account of the different forms of gender inequality over time, class and ethnic group" (Walby, 1990: 2). Patriarchal heritage and neo-patriarchal practices feed the procedural and symbolic violence of representation in the Mediterranean area. Patriarchy is a social system based on the exercise of male power but is also an interpretative key of the methods and justifications by means of which violence is exercised against women. It is inscribed within a repressive androcentric system. Patriarchy refers to a social system where power, authority, and material goods are concentrated in the hands of older men and whose transmission takes place through the male line, generally for the benefit of the first-born male patrilineal descendant: "patriarchy as a system of social structures and practices in which men dominate, oppress and exploit women" (Walby, 1990).

Patriarchalism is not, therefore, simply an interpretative category of violence referring to the economic, cultural, or religious peculiarities of actors of the past (Garcia-Moreno, Jansen, Ellsberg, Heise, & Watts, 2006). It is a complex key with which to interpret and justify, even today, the ambivalence of cultural influence and the opacity of multiple denigrating and segregating practices that involve women and men (Bartholini, 2019; Mackinnon, 2006; Volpato, 2011).

In the past, proof of this were honour crimes including female genital mutilation (FGM), forced marriages, early marriages, and, more recently, polygamy. Male supremacy is one of the oldest, most extensive, and most basic forms of power. As the *Manifesto REds.tockings* (1969) states, all other forms of exploitation and oppression (racism, capitalism, imperialism, etc.) are extensions of male supremacy, based originally on the control of sexuality and female reproduction. Biological, anatomical, and sexual differences are the discriminants used to exercise androcentric dominion. These are the elements preparatory to the construction of the subordinate, controlled, social, and cultural role of women. The sexual act which determines reproduction, and which is at the basis of the phenomenology of violence against women (VAW), is the act of male supremacy *par excellence*. All the cultural representations, which over time have arisen around it, perpetuate and underpin androcentric hegemony. Wherever the male sex was dominant, sexuality was considered in the West until recently, the exclusive prerogative of males as well as an instrument of female subjugation. It continues to be considered such in many other areas of the world. It has constituted a veritable "ordo rerum", the regulating principle of social relations between men and women based on the control of married women's fertility, and the virginity of those yet to marry (Lerner, 1986). Private patriarchy, as Walby argued, was replaced by patriarchy in the public sphere (Walby, 1990). Patriarchy claims that men, not women, have a right to be in control, can establish the rules, and should take priority over women. Although reproduction is a female prerogative, the exercise of reproduction has been assigned to self-legitimating male power, buttressed by uninterrupted cultural constructs aimed at creating appropriate representations for that purpose, confirming them over time through similar representations. Patriarchy actually contains a symbolic type of violence, legitimized implicitly by traditions, beliefs, and mechanisms of production and reproduction aimed at reconfirming gender asymmetries as well as appropriate representations meant to normalize and naturalize male domination. This is a symbolic kind of violence which makes women and the body of women one of many *provisions* available to men. At the same time, among their other *entitlements*, men have the right to the avail of the care, sexuality, and time of women as well as control over procreation, thanks to a mix of complicity, consensus, and acknowledgement (Morgan & Thapar-Björkert, 2006a) which sometimes involves the full consent of the women themselves. This binary situation of the sexes, perpetrated by ideological and religious conservatism, is a "situated" for of knowledge reflecting the views of hegemonic individuals and groups (Haraway, 1988). The Mediterranean area is still a place where relational modalities, attitudes, and communication codes referring to the symbolic universe of male domination prevail and create an organizational environment hostile to women. Lerner shows, for example, that veiling was introduced to distinguish between married (private) women and prostitutes (public women), between the marriage market (long-term relationships) and the "spot market" of short-lived liaisons (Hakim, 2015), as well as between the sexual and procreational meanings attributed to both classes of women.

This permits us to reflect on how ably androcentric universalism produces epistemic injustice through the construction of false truths and stereotyped images internalized by society (Friedan, 1963). Language and transmission of false truths facilitate both the subordination of women and male domination, above all, because "it needs to be highlighted that we live according to exclusively male genealogical systems. Our societies, constituted in equal parts by men and women, were generated by two genealogies, not by one: mothers/daughters and fathers/sons. Patriarchal power is organized through the subjection of one genealogy to another" (Irigaray, 1992: 15).

They are therefore hegemonic power relations established by patriarchy, intended as a device of authority and control, whose relations based on violence and subordination do not only concern the countries of the African continent but also the European ones because, as Corradi maintains, "The colonial matrix is active at geopolitical level towards Eastern Europe, Southern Italy, Greece, the Ottoman area" (Corradi & Connell, 2014: 30).

These are, above all constructs, based on the "honour and shame" a dyad which still emerges in relation to some crimes (honour killings, honour crimes) (Morgan & Thapar-Björkert, 2006a; Phillips, 2013), along with other forms of violence considered contiguous to it, like forced marriages and FGM, rooted in some of the family and community cultures of migrant groups. In this case, especially in some areas of Africa, the defence of family honour from the stain of shame still requires practices of multiple submission imposed by the hegemonic culture: modesty of body, pre-marital virginity, female marital fidelity, the use of the various kinds of veil, and the social obligation on the part of parents to prefer arranged marriages including those with very young brides. From public disapproval, critical judgment, and the right of veto certain customs we come to legal definitions of state authority (Razack, Smith, & Thobani, 2011) legitimizing the subordination of women in the name of patriarchy. Women who flee from Africa, however, and cross the Mediterranean are often not the victims of a sole perpetrator only. For them patriarchy assumes the contours not only of their fathers and husbands, but also of their traffickers, their recruiters and protectors, and, last but not least, of the regime of European borders which, by preventing their escape, rivets them to the condition of victim. A goodly number of women from Eastern Europe undergo similar consequences, where patriarchalism assumes the semblances of protection imposed coercive by contextual conditions and coaxed through the intimacy or proximity of the relationship.

In the Twenty-First century, patriarchal cultures and values persist in relation, precisely, to male interest which still seeks control over the sex trade and endeavours to maintain its historical dominance within the mating and marriage marts. It is not surprising, therefore, that the incidence of male sexual violence of all sorts has not diminished in modern societies.

Patriarchy is central to a comprehension not only of the sexual practices of recent past but also of social institutions and attitudes more in general, and their development in the twenty-first century.

One element that characterizes the contemporary migratory phenomenon is proximity violence of which women, in particular, are victims. The normalization of this kind of violence cannot be justified by the exceptionality of the migratory experience which cannot provide an exhaustive explanation of the dehumanization process to which this type of victim is subjected. As stated above, the real issue is that of identifying its aetiology in a cultural male- and patriarch-dominated regime. Individuals, whether knowingly or not, contribute to the production and reproduction of provisions and attitudes which actually normalize the violence which pervades their life cycles transversely, creating a "culture of violence" transmittable at intergenerational level (Siegel, 2013). As part of the legacy of a patriarchal culture, it has contributed to upholding "the established order, with its relationships of domination, its rights and abuses, its privileges and injustices" (Bourdieu, 1998: 7). Gender-based violence (GBV), in its symbolic makeup, is a phenomenon functional to the perpetuation of a system founded on "social constructs" (Berger & Luckmann, 1966) regarding the power relationships existing between men and women. That is, violence legitimized by a production of meaning that renders specific behavioural patterns and attitudes recognizable within situations or "domains of meaning", normalizing them at the same time. In the "reciprocal game of structures of relevance" (Schütz, 1956) an object or an event becomes the theme or the topic of a common mode of thought within a context that justifies and shares its meaning. From this perspective, proximity violence is a mode of expression, a product of masculine power confounded with it, while gender is a criterion bestowing order on reality. The cultural paradigm of patriarchy brings together all the originally ill-negotiated, divergent forms of polyculturalism, legitimizes male hegemony, and justifies violence with a view to maintaining the balance within the family, intact.

For a long time, patriarchy was the maintenance device of the symbolic violence "implicitly legitimised by traditions, beliefs and the mechanisms producing and reproducing the practices involved in the renegotiation of asymmetries and representations used to normalise and naturalise male domination" (Bartholini, 2016: 75). It should be seen as a survival of the archaic world, relegated to the past, yet, even today, traces of patriarchalism resurface (Garcia-Moreno et al., 2006) which, though common opinion attributes them to newcomers to Europe, actually re-exhume justifications of models that have not been totally dismissed from Mediterranean cultures.

In a patriarchal view of the dynamics of relationships, bodies are subjected to violence in that they are seen as bearers of shame and dishonour. As shame is the negative counterpart of honour, it is closely linked to ways in which different cultures interpret and evaluate honour (Herzfeld, 1980). The research on Kabila cosmology which first appeared in a volume by Peristiany (1965), and later taken up by Pierre Bourdieu in his Masculine Domination (1998), revolves around the issue of male honour and the link between the public reputation of men and the private virtue of women, to focus on the persistence of practices and meanings which place women and men in a specular position and can be used today to interpret symbolic violence and maintain the illusion of claims of female emancipation and equal opportunities (Bimbi & Basaglia, 2013). The honour-shame dyad generally characterizes premodern or archaic societies marked by a "bond of reason and emotion transforming the body of the victim into matter to be moulded" (Bimbi, 2015: 74).

1.3 Dehumanization, Objectification, and Reification of the Migrant Woman's Body

Segregation is a practice typical of patriarchal systems, one which tends to place the weakest subject in a position of permanent subordination. One of its consequences is exposure of the segregated subjects to the possibility of being violated. In order for this to happen materially, a process of dehumanization needs to be carried out by the perpetrator(s) in order to create in the victim a type of alienation based on an ineliminable sense of inferiority and powerlessness. In the 1960s, Fanon (1961) held that this condition of self-depreciation, self-immobilization by the victim was a consequence of the colonial oppression of subordinates by hegemonic groups. However, the process to which we refer here is not definable in terms of groups but as an inherent aspect of interpersonal dynamics which spill over into broader contexts. It is a personal condition reflecting the disavowal of others by limiting the victim's chances of emancipating herself from the perpetrator.

Tajfel used the more appropriate term "dehumanization" (Tajfel, 1981) to indicate the preliminary practice required by the perpetrator to exploit the victim's body. This means that the perpetrator does not consider the woman a person, but one of the many objects he can avail himself of to exert power which is actually wielded starting from the asymmetry of patriarchal cultures and grounded in the subordination of one gender to the other. We might, therefore, consider dehumanization as one of the extreme consequences of the gender asymmetry present in patriarchal cultures.

Asymmetry between the victim and the perpetrator produces a gap between what, for the perpetrator, is human and what is not, a gap, therefore, between those endowed with the prototypical qualities of humanness and those believed to lack them. Dehumanization posits, a priori, denial of humanity, gender humanity, for example, thus permitting the exploitation of the victim by means of practices made possible by the physical proximity or occupation of the body in a shared environment. Dehumanization permits the objectifying subject to approach the objectified one, allowing the former to exploit or exert power over the latter, something that differentiates this form of violence from others, like rape, for example, which imply the non-permanence of the victim. In an attempt to define this process better, we might point out that objectification permits evaluation of the objectified person using parameters related to objects, commodities, denying the human traits of the person in question, thus dehumanizing her/him. "Objectifying" attitudes are oriented towards sexual or material functions as a source of labour separated from the other components of a person's identity and considered in isolation as a representation of the whole person. In other words, it is a phenomenon which depersonalizes the human being, appraising it on the basis of a part of the self alone, in this case, the sexual body or the body to be exploited for labour, ignoring every other aspect. The vulnerability of the victim (Kirby, 2006), on the one hand, is a characterizing aspect of gender segregation and, on the other, a *conditio* sine qua non which permits the exploitation of another for personal or collective purposes. It precedes all forms of violence and is enhanced by conditions of abuse. Violence perpetrated against a woman's body affects her vulnerability by disabling her very chances of self-defence.

The dehumanization process is a particularly significant risk when it comes to the majority of migrants, precisely because of the interweave of exogenous and endogenous factors characterizing their lives. It does not concern asymmetry of power alone but the social scene within which it is constructed. In the case of migrant women, there are three variables: their material living conditions which make them vulnerable in terms of everyday life; the subjective dimension which exposes some of them more readily to violence; and situations of temporary difficulty which develop gradually, aggravating their already precarious condition.

If, historically speaking, denial of the humanity of others served exclusively to justify exploitation, degradation, and violence, today the practices of dehumanization testified by thousands of victims of migratory violence imply that the victims themselves adhere to the very project which erodes their humanity in a very subtle manner. Dehumanization, accompanied by depersonalization which ranks individuals according to their belongingness, ethnicity, village, and gender, of course, facilitates this process. When several indicators, like being female, a foreigner, and poor intersect when defining a person, the result of this process is, for the most part, taken for granted.

In cases of ethnic war or trafficking, the term that best describes the dynamics that produce dehumanization and favour prostitution, for example, is de-individualization (Fanon, 1961). According to Fanon, the colonized experience a condition of alienation based on irreparable feelings of inferiority produced by devaluation of the culture to which they belong and the imposition of alien values. Thus, a progressive weakening of personal identity is brought about by practices and actions with which the colonized are not seen as specific, identifiable, responsible entities but as a confused, anonymous, amorphous, aggregate (Volpato, 2013). Dehumanization, depersonalization, and de-individualization converge to contribute to the process of objectification. The latter unites the previous processes to a point where the individual is thought of and treated as an object, a tool, a commodity. Martha Nussbaum (2011) divides this process of objectification into seven parts:

1. Instrumentality: the object as a tool exploited by others.
2. Denial of autonomy: the object as an entity deprived of autonomy and self-determination.
3. Inertia: the object as an entity lacking the ability to act and be active.
4. Fungibility: the object considered as being interchangeable with other objects belonging to the same category.
5. Violability: the object as an entity devoid of boundaries capable of guaranteeing its integrity whereby it may be torn to pieces.
6. Property: the object belongs to someone and can, therefore, be sold, bought, or hired.
7. Denial of subjectivity: the object as an entity whose experiences and feelings are negligible.

For MacKinnon "women live in sexual objectification like fish in water" (1989: 124). Objectification represents a reiterated experience in certain environments and contexts from which it is impossible to escape precisely because of the pervasiveness of its effects. Sexual exploitation is a product – perhaps the most common – of a kind of objectification which stems from a successful dehumanization procedure based on processes of social categorization, sanctioning the segregation of individuals – the most vulnerable – from the human community.

To separate discourse regarding violence from the normative and cultural constructs that justify it would be tantamount to severing it from its classifications which would lead, in turn, to a sort of "racialization" of behaviour patterns (Crenshaw, 1991; Razack et al., 2011). If, in actual fact, the terms "honour" and "shame" do not appear in the everyday discourse of western societies, the view that family honour represents a cultural aspect operating only within given traditional contexts of immigration is not credible. The decline in judgment criteria based on honour and chastity and replaced by those of human dignity and the inalienable rights of the person are disproved by hard fact. On the contrary, honour and shame have re-emerged as social attitudes and sentiments to be fostered (Appiah, 2010; Turnaturi, 2012), even in modern ethics. Shame, in particular, seems to have assumed positive connotations for the formation of a public ethic of dignity, integrity, modesty, decency (Nussbaum, 2000).

In the European and international debate, honour and shame are considered the basis of patriarchy and typical of a late-archaic, as opposed to a modern, system of reputation, defined according to the following three contrary dyads:

1. Patriarchal family and blood relations as opposed to family-by-choice and non-ascribed relational networks.
2. Homogeneity between the vital worlds of private and public life as opposed to pluralization and the individualization of universes of meaning.
3. A propensity to preserve tradition as opposed to an inclination to anticipate change.

The representation of the irreconcilability of practices and meanings, related to different family models, as entities incorporated in the cultures of traditional groups, or typical of late-modern societies, emerges today in particular, as a result of migration processes and within a framework of transition towards new geopolitical orders.

Bourdieu's paradigm ends up by favouring segregationist practices and contributing, to some extent, to the exoticization of harmful practices, while "our" violence is seen as a residue of social pathologies that we are overcoming. The phenomena of marriage markets, child brides, the outdoor prostitution of Nigerian women (Peano, 2013), or genital mutilation, are some of the aspects of a segregationist and patriarchal type of culture. The risk, however, is that they be reabsorbed within an everyday, destinal dimension of migratory cultures, placing vulnerability and resistance by the victims "other than us" on the same plane, without evaluating the power of suggestion and possible instances of cross-fertilization implemented within host-country contexts.

This is because gender violence is, above all, structural (Farmer, 2003), characterized by norms, attitudes, and stereotypes diffused within the ambits of the "world of life" and institutional environments.

Confronting definitions of violence means confronting European cultural models belonging to a past and as yet not dismissed, which resurface along with the migratory flows and which it is necessary to recognize starting from signs of the widespread dehumanization of victims of gender violence.

1.4 The Opaque Connections Between "Violence Against Women" and "Gender Violence"

For several decades now, the subject of VAW stands at the intersection between social and cultural phenomena, an understanding of which permits us to intercept some of the extensive transformations late-modern scenarios are undergoing in Europe and, more generally, in the west. Although initially monopolized by feminist literature (De Beauvoir, 1949; Mitchell, 1984), the topic now traverses multiple fields of analysis. If, on the one hand, the phenomenon involves different sectors of society, such as the family, the workplace, systems of coexistence between groups belonging to different cultures, etc., on the other it is analysed from many dissimilar disciplinary perspectives.

These perspectives converge on the essential elements which characterize it: male domination, asymmetry of roles, but also the vulnerability of the victim and the proximity indicators of self-acceptance put into practice by the victims themselves: resistance and resilience.

These regard rapports between subjects involved in power relations which orient analyses of the phenomenon in two directions: the oppression men exert over women by means of the hierarchization of difference (Bartholini, 2019; Bartky, 1990; Bimbi & Basaglia, 2013) within specific contexts; confirmation of the existence of rigid confines between gender identities (Bimbi, 2015; Connell, 2002) based on cultural prejudices and mental constructs rooted in and endorsed by the social groups in which they are evident. GBV and VAW are often used interchangeably, since most GBV is perpetrated by men against women. Even the expressions used are not univocal although VAW and GBV are undoubtedly the linguistic periphrases which best describe the aspects peculiar to the phenomenon.

The use of the term gender violence is recent and dates back to 1995, when the fourth United Nations Conference was held in Beijing in 1995. Its use was born from the need to emphasize the existence of subjectivity until then destined to social subordination (Bimbi, 2012).

The Council of Europe Convention on preventing and combatting VAW, the so-called Istanbul Convention (2011), besides defining one and the other as violations of human rights, also indicated its range of action within the spheres of public and the private life alike.

It represents an exemplary model as a process of evolution, still in progress, characterized by key concepts such as: participation of civil society; support of the organizations and authorities in charge of regulatory enforcement; role of information and communication; regulatory harmonization and international cooperation.

However, it is above all Article 3 of the Istanbul Convention, consisting of 81 articles divided into twelve chapters and preceded by a Preamble to report a series of fundamental definitions:

For the purposes of this Convention:

(a) The expression "violence against women" means a violation of human rights and a form of discrimination against women, including all acts of violence based on gender that cause or are likely to cause harm or suffering of physical, sexual, psychological, or economic nature, including threats to perform such acts, coercion or arbitrary deprivation of liberty, both in public and private life.
(b) The term "domestic violence" means all acts of physical, sexual, psychological, or economic violence that occur within the family or family unit or between current or previous spouses or partners, regardless of whether the perpetrator of these acts, he shares or has shared the same residence with the victim.
(c) The term "gender" refers to roles, behaviour, activities, and socially constructed attributes that a given society considers appropriate for women and men.

(d) The expression "gender-based violence against women" means any violence directed against a woman as such, or which affects women disproportionately.
(e) "Victim" means any natural person who suffers the acts or behaviour referred to in paragraphs (a) and (b) above.
(f) The term "women" also means girls under the age of 18.

The VAW paradigm is rooted in a comprehensive understanding of the phenomenon of violence based on masculine domination and patriarchy over women, perceived and treated as inferior parts of the society (Merry, 2009). The second paradigm is better understood in the development of an ecological model/approach (Casique & Furegato, 2006) which accounts for diverse, intersected dimensions among personal, situational, and contextual factors. Despite their being interwoven, they need to be considered differently in relation to the variegated spectrum of situations and relationships which underscore the phenomenon both in the north-west and the rest of the world (Kapur, 2002). In the case of the first of these two – VAW – the emphasis is placed almost by accident on the rhetoric of power based on male dominance within gender relations, the abuse of power exerted by men over women as an effect of the "androcentric role" they play (Bourdieu, 1998).

VAW is perpetrated by men "as the dominant group" in order to maintain the advantages they derive from being dominant (Bartholini, 2013; Collins, 2008; Corradi, 2009; Romito, 2000) availing themselves of "naturalized" abuse of devices of power and bio-power (Foucault, 1976), which even go so far as to arrive at the dehumanization of the victim. The expression violence against women refers, therefore, to ascertained biological and historical subalternity, stable even in the tireless reproduction of its practices. As sanctioned by the recommendations made by international bodies, it does not endorse neutral definitions referring to generic theoretical positions. Instead it is an effect of cultural representations sedimented over time, which originally served to "make the unusual customary" (Moscovici, 1984: 49) and turned into concrete experiences and modes of behaviour after a series of adjustments carried out to normalize and concretize what formerly seemed abstract. It identifies a macro-group of people vulnerable by definition – women – and outlines the binary and asymmetric dimension of male domination (Bourdieu, 1998), traceable back to customary norms and notions of morality and masculine values, as well as to religious beliefs, to practices passed down through history. It is a modus vivendi that knows no geographical boundaries and rests on beliefs which in Europe, by way of example, tolerated honour killings at length, while in large areas of the rest of the world FGM (BMBF 2009; WHO 2002), forced marriages, and stoning (WHO 2002, 2005) are still authorized. These are all forms of violence practised to the detriment of women by the ethnic group or state to which they belong, as well as by their families themselves, a fact bearing witness to widespread cultural legitimation of violence.

The second definition makes the positions of those who perpetrate violence and those who are oppressed by it explicit also from a symbolic point of view. It refers to violence exercised against "a" more vulnerable gender, where violence "is directed against a woman because she is a woman or [...] affects women disproportionately" (Istanbul Convention, 2011) within a sex-gender system where the male occupies the predominant position (Rubin, 1997). GBV includes violence against men, boys, and sexual minorities or those with nonconforming gender identities. However, this emphasis acknowledges the heightened vulnerability of females from childhood throughout their lifecycle and the profound, long-term impacts of sexual and physical violence on women and girls throughout their lives. GBV is a widespread and systematic violation of fundamental human rights violations and an enduring form of gender-based discrimination. It occurs in every country of the world, rich and poor, stable and in conflict, and affects most women and girls, regardless of their age or socio-economic status. GBV is a term used to describe any harmful act that is perpetrated against a person's will, and that is based on socially ascribed differences between males and females. While men and boys can be victims/survivors of some types of GBV (particularly sexual violence) around the world, GBV has a greater impact on women and girls. Gender associated with the topic of violence becomes, primarily, an analytical category used to interpret social changes and differences between cultures. So, firstly, the stereotypes, ideologies, behaviours, and lifestyles conventionally associated with feminine and masculine vary considerably from one culture to another. Secondly, "women and men are not universal and unalterable essences, but rather specific existences, changing far from uniform" (Fernandez-Alvarez, 2014: 48). In defining the GBV, it becomes clear that any violence perpetrated against a weaker subject is regulated by the principle of normative heterosexuality which is performatively hegemonic (Preciado, 2014). Historically acknowledged gender segregation between masculinity and femininity lies at the basis of practices leading to the violation of women, LGBTs, and men in conditions of vulnerability. Examples of GBV throughout the lifecycle include (but are not limited to): sex-selective abortion, differential access to food and services, sexual exploitation and abuse, including trafficking, child marriage, female genital mutilation/cutting, sexual harassment, dowry/bride price abuse, honour killing, domestic or intimate partner violence, deprivation of inheritance or property, and elder abuse. As such, VAW is one type of GBV, in which the gender difference favours violence against people who – as women and homosexuals but also foreigners, the elderly, children – are in an asymmetrical and weakened position with respect to their perpetrators. Therefore, most of the violence is favoured by the person's attributes – "I am a child", "I am a foreigner", "I am an elderly person" – to which is added the gender aggravating factor when the victim itself is not already a homosexual or more often a woman. Gender and violence are a binomial defining the identity of the victims and the perpetrators, but which can be enlarged to cover the entire issue of gender violence, leaving, however, the dominant role of the male intact. This causes views of gender to focus on roles perceived and played according to the expectations of scripts repeated over time and space, which denote the constant in the rapport between perpetrators and victims as "a fluctuating artifice, a ceaseless motion in action, a practice of improvisation within a scene of constraint which does not deny the violence but rather presumes it" (Butler, 2004: 26), acting in a way to impose a representation as congenial as possible to the will of the perpetrator.

In both of the above-described semantic contexts, violence involves some form of social exclusion, public discrimination (Crisp, Morris, & Refstie, 2012; Jaji, 2009) secondary victimization (Pinelli, 2011; Tognetti & Rossi 2016), exploitation of labour (Coin, 2004), forced prostitution (Krause-Vilmar, 2011; Nagguja et al., 2014; Peano, 2013), and sexual abuse (Arbel, Dauvergne, & Millbank, 2014; Crisp et al., 2012).

Although recent literature defines gender violence as the exercise of physical and psychological dominance over a victim and foregrounds the various modalities (direct, indirect, physical, symbolic, cultural, instrumental, etc.), of which it avails itself explicitly, the problem remains confined within a cultural paradigm which tolerates gender inequality, even when it does not legitimate it. Gender violence not only acts upon bodies but also through bodies, in a combination which is frequently complicit and consensual but also devoid of acknowledgement (Morgan & Thapar-Björkert, 2006b). In this sense, gender violence is a "modernist phenomenon" (Corradi, 2009 and following), that is, one which is attributable to cultural models of the past that refer to codifications of inter-gender relationships availing themselves of stereotypes and representations of patriarchal inter-sex structures. However, while VAW incontrovertibly describes the exercise and abuse of the power of men over women, GBV fails to conceal widespread gender subalternity to the male. In actual fact, it validates said subalternity by taking for granted that the diversities inherent to the gender subjected to violence are naturally associable to practices of segregation and labelling (Morgan & Thapar-Björkert, 2006b). It finds legitimacy in the power relationship between genders where the disvalue consists in the fact of being different from, other than, the dominant male.

Even legal rulings have adopted this kind of division which polarizes women or genders. In an incontrovertible way, Art.1 of the General Recommendation No. 19, of the 11th session of the United Nations, defined VAW as a form of "gender-based" discrimination, "like that violence directed to a person on the basis of his/her gender". This article also included acts inflicting physical, mental, or sexual damage or suffering, threats of similar action, coercion, and other deprivation of liberty. The convention of Istanbul, too, defined it as "any violence directed against a woman as such, or affecting women in a disproportionate way" (article 3) as gender-type violence.

In conclusion, the term GBV undermines the binary juxtaposition of "men and women", as perpetrators and victims. It widens the plethora of victims by confirming the principle of male hegemonic heteronormativity. The number of subjectivities to be considered, therefore, expands horizontally, but GBV does not define the epistemological core which permits the exercise of violence. It does not reveal the decisive principle that explains violent action and violent ritual, as well as the dramaturgy of violence.

1.5 Proximity Violence, Bodies, and Emotions

Following the international legal framework on VAW or GBV, what appears, however, to be explored to a lesser degree are the mechanisms that make it possible to continue a violent relationship, whereby traditional categories like "gender", "power", and "domain" prove insufficient. The gender violence experienced during migration throws considerable light on the comprehension of the mechanisms permitting to explain its genesis and its reproduction.

We argue in the following pages that this kind of VAW or GBV is specific, distinct, and that, as that it belongs to the realm of proximity relationships, we may well define it as violence of proximity. In similar relationships, the authorized-proximus is not a "neutral subject", but the person most intimate and closest to the victim at emotional and life-plan level. Upon the emotional plane we find the dynamics of trust, sentimental closeness, or psychological oppression which determine acceptance of violence on the part of the victim. The hope of a better future is used as a lever by the perpetrator to coerce the victim to accept the present while waiting a possible better future. The violence suffered by the victim is produced also from resistance by the victim to admit the plight in which she finds herself.

Proximity violence precedes gender violence and/or VAW at both theoretical-reflection and extrinsic-phenomenic levels. It constitutes the architrave of the phenomenological spectrum which makes it possible to grasp its substantially different aspects while, at the same time, placing itself beyond the forms of violence examined in the preceding paragraphs. In the pages that follow, we shall sustain that the type of violence found in acts against women is of a particular kind, made possible only because the perpetrator enjoys a special type of habitual proximity with the victim for reasons of *jus sanguinis* (a father or a close relative), because of being a *coniugo* (partner) or due to a *causa simulandi* (that is simulation whereby the perpetrator "makes believe", "pretends"). Both the proximity violence perpetrated by right of blood or by conjugal right belong to the cultural bedrock of patriarchy and considered "a woman's destiny". Proximity violence perpetrated because of *causa simulandi* is a degeneration of the former because it incorporates justifications typical of a patriarchal system accompanied by manipulation of the victims and pretence by means of which immunity and rights over the victim are acquired with the consensus of the victim herself. In these situations, the perpetrator is not either an extraneous or neutral subject but contextually "the" person or "one of the" persons legitimized by the victim herself within whose sphere of influence and under whose dominion she places herself. This happens by virtue of the material and symbolic oppression experienced by the more vulnerable subject and which convinces her of the necessity/opportunity to delegate the very possibility of existing to another. This delegation is attenuated by the victim's trust in her persecutor, something which precedes the perpetration of violence and induces her to accept the situation. The hypothesis whereby trust is at the root of the perpetration of violence and its emergence as an action of coercion and domestication appears reasonable to us, if accompanied by two corollaries:

1. At times the vulnerability of victims borders on sentimental dependence which turns into resistance against acknowledgement of the abuse to which they are subjected. Within relationships ensconced in the private and the sentimental, it is easier for the weaker subject to become the object of violence. She not only connotes the relationship but also provides the humus of the ordinary practice upon which the rules of play between the victim and perpetrator rest (Gagnon, 2004). The objective of its implementation is to weaken the victim, by working on her vulnerability, until preventive remission of any form of rebellion is achieved. The expectation of violence is part of the hot emotions which are at once rhythmic and strongly entraining and induce the victim to expose herself to them. It is, therefore, a matter of "forward panic" (Collins, 2008), like that which spurs soldiers into battle, urging those whose lives are in danger to move forward and face danger directly, instead of fleeing.
2. At times, hope in a better future is used as leverage by the perpetrator to oblige the victim to accept present adverse conditions as a necessary part of a personal plan aimed at improving her material conditions. Furthermore, Bernstein (2007) and Illouz (2007) have provided ample proof of the progressive intrusion of the logic of commerce into sexual relations. This kind of logic becomes shareable often within dynamics managed by those who claim ownership of the female body favoured by emotional dependence used as a cementing agent between the victim and the perpetrator.

The underlying theme is that of continuous "testing" of the "intimate contract" by passive resistance on the part of the victim and the consequent opportunity of continuous renewal of consent towards a modality of hetero-management of her very existence. The violence endured is itself the outcome of dependence/resistance by the victim, unable to sever the dynamic ties that make her the perpetrator's prey. Male domination and the way in which it is not only imposed but subjected to is paradoxical subjection, the effect of what Bourdieu called symbolic violence.

We might define GBV more analytically as a form of "proximity violence found within interpersonal ties, where it is the Weberian-matrix-like affective action itself that constitutes the unreasonable justification of its implementation" (Bartholini 2013 and following).

As a phenomenon that is particularly adaptable within relations characterized by temporal continuity and spatial closeness, it substantiates behavioural dynamics based on oppression, claims of recognition of identity, and attempts at ritualizing violence itself.

Proximity violence is, therefore, the litmus test of a category whose defining criteria are provided by the various arenas into which we may divide public discourse. This is not only because of the problem that it represents in itself but due to its priorities of legitimate consideration, its practical implications, its theoretical references, and the side-issues upon which it borders or at times even crosses in its entirety. It traces its karstic sources back to a more artfully constructed patriarchal dimension and presents devices of power linked to a single kind of public discourse, supported also by globalized migrations which have led to co-influence – sometimes at a distance – cultures based on substantial, original *Male Domination* (Bourdieu, 1998).

It is precisely migrations and the cultural "customs clearances" that accompany them, that normalize the violence experienced during the journey not only by migrant women but by minors, LGBTs, and young men too, which highlight some biases. The first of these stems from the fact of having taken for granted the end of male hegemony as a result of female emancipation and having considered violent phenomena as mere regurgitations of pre-modern conditions that have no place in the present. The second is attributable to attempts at separating discourse on violence from the construction of norms in defence of the victimized female body and from scientific approaches to the care of relational distress. The third is found in the self-referential representation of the west as advanced, stable, pacified (Butler, 2008), and underestimation of the multiple forms used by symbolic violence to reproduce itself (Bourdieu, 1998).

The social phenomenon of proximity violence, in its gender displays (Goffman, 1976) and in its public representations, refers to narrative devices capable of legitimizing or contrasting political discourse and decisions within the ambit of policies concerning proximity gender violence.

Besides the matter of the size of the phenomenon in terms of prevalence and incidence, themes and issues remain open as regards the social construction of violence, its incorporation into the habitus of men and women, the persistence of mechanisms of domination expressed by the subjectivity of the victims, that is, through mental constructs such as their categories of perception and evaluation.

Furthermore, there exists a level of violence deemed unlawful that is perpetrated within a given society, and there is violence committed or carried out silently. The boundaries between them are not only difficult to plot but they also generate several interdependencies and procedural subterfuges capable of revealing and concealing them. Variables such as age, status, income, education, social background, self-perception, and self-definition, even when considering composite incidences of sexual and gender elements that identify perpetrators and victims of violence within a specific reference context, are not sufficient to describe the multiple intersections that sustain gender violence. Above all, they lose sight of the implicit effects that derive from them when codifying gender relations. The data provided by the Italian statistics office, Istat's 2014 survey and the previous Urban project (Basaglia, Lotti, Misiti, & Tola, 2007) reveal the existence and persistence in Italy of value systems and social constructs that include levels of acceptance of violence by women who have experienced it. From this point of view, in-depth investigation of the modalities of perception and tolerance of violence acquires crucial significance. A recent report by the European Commission (Gracia & Lila, 2015) reveals that, among other things, a small though significant sector of interviewees (including young people and victims) tends to acknowledge the existence of violent behaviour, underlining the fact of how attitudes of acceptance and tolerance are still quite widespread (ibidem), transversal, and persistent at inter-generational level. After the research Urban carried out over a decade ago (Basaglia et al., 2007) into the perception of VAW using gender-culture oriented markers, involving both the general population (women and men) and operatives within dedicated sectors, no further research was carried out at national level in Italy to document the cultural background and the systems of social representations which structure and justify violent behaviour and the radicalization of women-men role stereotypes. Furthermore, the investigations carried out over the past five years in Europe, with the exception of the abovementioned report, are still fragmentary, inhomogeneous, and poorly developed, especially in Italy, something which denotes a lack of specific scientific investigations of questions of attitude.

It is not a matter, therefore, of defining a "one-size-fits-all" approach capable of dealing with such a multifaceted, complex, and all-pervasive phenomenon. It is a question of loosening some of the knots and identifying the extreme ends of the cultural continuum existing between men and women. This, in order to show how the analytical category of explicit violence, differences in violent phenomenology, diverse representations addressed by *vetero* – and neo-patriarchal cultures, indigenous and migrant – mutually reinforce each other as a result of migratory flows. It is also necessary to point out that violence is not exclusively about women but about "genders" and is associated with other indicators and, lastly, that proximity violence implies that "neighbours" are people who are close to the victim.

The term "*proximus* closest" derives from a Latin absolute superlative indicating "the person closest to another", and may refer to a type of relationship where the subjects are linked, in a spatiotemporal dimension, permitting physical contiguity and exploitation of the victim. The *proximus* is the other who, in a rapport of physical proximity, occupies a dominant position (Bartholini, 2013, 2016). As this dominance is almost always explicitly founded on gender difference, on direct and indirect physical and psychological abuse of the victim, perpetrated in a temporal *dureé*, it may be deemed to belong to the category of proximity. The *durée* indicates the time of the biographical experience and that is different from the chronological time. The time in which the one – the victim - and the other – perpetrator- recognizes themselves in the proximity relationship, recognizes and accepts their mutual roles.

The category of proximity, which illuminates the intimate character of the relationship, makes violence within the victim-perpetrator dyad and the exploitation of the victim outside the relationship too (as in the case of sexual exploitation) possible.

Gender itself may, therefore, be considered "a fluctuating artifice, an incessant work in progress, a practice of improvisation within a scenario of constraint, which does not recuse violence but presupposes it" (Butler, 2004) within a mechanism of proximity. Gender is a variable favouring proximity violence which, however, does not justify it completely.

The bond of trust between the victim and the perpetrator permits the exercise of proximity violence. The violence exercised by a stranger would result in a defensive reaction from the victim. Unlike GBV, proximity violence is based on a pact made precisely within a relationship that opacifies instrumental rationality and blurs exploitation within fiduciary bonds. Proximity violence is constitutive of the relationship, self-sufficient, self-immune, and excludes conflict. This violence is tolerated and almost shared. There is no conflict between victim and perpetrator, but subjection and acceptance by the victim who does not rebel precisely because of the very proximity link.

1. Violence is both a tool for regulating relationships and an autonomous social force capable of giving meaning to reality. As a structuring force in the relationship, it gives participants tasks and roles within a commercial pact that has essential emotional values in binding contractors.
2. Because violence – in different forms and in different ways – becomes the bond itself of the relationship, it assumes the characteristics of self-sufficiency. In other words, violence is "enough" to keep the relationship going.
3. The relationship based on violence excludes any other form of internal resistance to violence, which becomes indispensable for maintenance of the relationship, thus making it self-immune.

Separating the discourse on proximity violence from the patriarchal representations that justify it, as well as from the processes of vulnerability and resistance in place, would, therefore, mean separating it from any possible interpretation that "naturalizes" it, and this would produce a sort of "racialization" of the migrants (Crenshaw, 1991; Razack et al., 2011). This would suggest that only migrants, due to a patriarchal culture, different from that of the West, normalized relations of proximal violence: rape, genital mutilation, marriage markets of child brides, sexual exploitation, etc., would be the product of behaviours attributable to particular ethnic groups or races.

As far as the victim is concerned, the perpetrator is in an asymmetrical, prevaricating position. From this point of view, the possibility of carrying out violence is subordinate to the behaviour and deeds of the perpetrator who dominates the victim who finds herself in a condition of absolute vulnerability due to the situation.

1.6 The Ritual of Proximity Violence

Contemporary violence has assumed characteristics that are specific compared to pre-modern violence that had mostly physical and collective connotations. Postmodernist violence, on the other hand, is proximal, that is, it is intimate and close to the other-than-self. It is multiple, meaning physical and symbolic, material and immaterial, and its main location is within intimate relationships. It is a form of violence rooted in interpersonal ties. This is a new type of violence consisting in a dual identity; on the one hand, it has a structural dimension based on the universal disparity of man–woman power relations, on the other hand, it possesses a constitutive dimension which involves the establishment of the relationship by adopting strategies and procedures that lead to spontaneous acceptance of the relationship itself. GBV, in its proximal form, is the "product of a set of markers that ritualise the eruption of emotional energy aimed at maintaining deviant relationships between the partners who are close, that is, not strangers to each other. Proximity comprises mutual acceptance of the physical and symbolic positions of the subjects involved. It implies that a physical space of a relational nature is determined by the limits which, in the reticular and functional structure relating each element with all the others, acquire their spatial expressions within the boundaries that frame it. Proximity violence takes form within a field of strong emotional tension between the victim and her proximus" (Bartholini, 2013).

This kind violence may be considered, therefore, is the axis instituting the relationship, a substratum within a context characterized by a high degree of oppression, a context from which the actors involved find it very hard to free themselves. In this context, males who fail to receive recognition within the public sphere tend to turn themselves into the personification of the abuser within the private sphere, perpetrating forms of violence against the other. The inability of the contemporary male to accept the partial nature of his role turns the strategy of conflict into the intrinsic bearer of clashes as well as of confrontation, causing practices of violence to erupt. These form the basis of relationships aimed at achieving authentic redemption of identity (Bartholini 2013 and following).

Consuelo Corradi has proposed a three-dimensional structure of micro, meso, and macro levels of violence extensively (Corradi, 2009). The first level regards situations that arise within the dynamics of interpersonal relations between perpetrators and victims; the second refers to social roles and networks; finally, the third level concerns the community involved and social policies.

Specific, dynamic interactional situations belong to the first level (micro-social) regarding the two parties involved and concern:

- The characteristics of situations that generate violence such as a person's ritual interaction and specific communicative framework.
- A strong emotional tension attributable to causes internal to the relationship and having peculiar modes of expression.
- Profiling the perpetrator.
- Victim/perpetrator dynamics.

At the meso-social level, both roles and types of family networks are considered on the basis of:

- The socio-economic characteristics of the subjects involved as well as their age, citizenship, and type of occupation.
- The roles they play within partnership or family systems.
- Gender roles.

At the third and final level (macro-social), the issue concerns:

- The community to which those involved belong (neighbourhood, ethnic community, district network) which protects or is indifferent to them.
- The threshold of tolerance of specific violent events inside and outside the proximity relationship.
- Law enforcement policies and reception services.

In this final paragraph of this first chapter, we shall focus, in particular, on the first of these three dimensions, that is, on the micro-social dimension of victim–

perpetrator relationships, in the belief that this level intersects with the others in a play of reflecting mirrors.

Proximity violence may be considered like the staging of a veritable theatrical ritual where emotional energy is emitted from within an oppressive context.

This is an acknowledged ritual, a sort of frame capable of attributing meaning to experiences, of framing everyday situations bestowing meaning on interactions. Proximity violence is both a frame and a framework which fabricates situations by multiplying them indefinitely and providing them with different interpretative keys (keying) while maintaining the original script. A key is an aspect of the framework: while the frame permits the situation to be framed, identifying the framework which provides logical interpretations to the events underlined by the key granting "access" to the situation and permitting one to grasp the implications and nuances implicit in it and, where necessary, shifting to the visual angle from which to interpret the situation.

If framing regards the positioning of the actors within a context, keying leads to the identification of the responsibilities and the causes which trigger the event/action (Goffman, 1974). Each culture is based on a limited set of fundamental models for the interpretation of everyday situations. Therefore, culture is itself a framework of frameworks, that is, a set of shared interpretative schemata, a shared symbolic structure, to which real forms of social organization correspond. From this angle, proximity violence acts as a primary framework, since proximity violence is not inherent to a situation but constitutes it. It is interesting to observe, from our point of view, that a person's ability to adapt to a given frame is not innate but acquired and requires that the experience obtained within the situation be mirrored or reflected within that of broader contexts. It constitutes an act of concrete adaptation to reality on the part of all those mutually linked by the same experiences within the same space-time congeries. Frames can be transformed through keying, a process by which certain activities can be defined in different ways. This is how proximity violence is interpreted, made necessary, and legitimized, therefore. Proximity violence – not "gender-violence" or "violence against women" – is reiterative and totally inherent in relationships that are peculiar each one in its own way. The victim, however, is not born a victim, and, above all, often victims do not always consider themselves victims or are they deemed such by their communities or contexts.

If observed at a micro-social level, that is, in face-to-face exchanges between men and women, violence arises within a field of strong emotional tension. Proximity violence includes emotions like anger, fear, humiliation, shame, erotic attraction, possessiveness, and frustration. It is never "cold" but occurs in a crescendo of forms and mode of behaviour (verbal confrontation, threats, beatings, etc.) that precedes the final furious explosion. Its very dynamics are a chain of interactions, a series of socially legitimized situational rituals justifying them, a frame within which two behavioural patterns recur: attack in an outburst of emotion having an oppressive routine of a before and an after; a duration, a *durée*. *Durée* indicates a continuous succession of violent acts; but, above all, it describes the cause-effect process unfolding the deeds performed by the subjects involved in the violent action and in a temporal perception which is, at once, an inter-subjective aspect of the relationship and of the collective or "prospective" plane of the interacting subjects intertwined in each other's experiences (Bartholini 2013). To put it briefly, the exercise of violence occurs between subjects who are also workers, members of other groups, neighbours, etc. They possess an identity which is acknowledged or scorned within the public sphere. Oppression and temporal *durée* make violence and its sedimentation possible, ritualizing it as a constitutive trait of intimacy.

The production of emotion becomes the very condition of the violent structure of the relationship. In some ways, violence is contiguous to eroticism because both relational conditions are riddled with a surplus of emotional energy. From this angle – violence-eroticism – Randall Collins's position proves interesting. At the centre of this hypothesis stand the concepts of "ritual" and "situation". The latter as a unit by which to analyse non-random actions which, if associated with symbolic outcomes, become ritual.

All situations have their own peculiar rules and processes that make each one different from all others, making each ritual potentially specific. The possibility of transforming a situation depends on how symbols are managed and shared and what emotional level is reached to unfold the interactions between the subjects involved so that they turn into what Goffman calls "ritual interaction", underlining the coagulating potential deriving from raising the emotional thresholds (mutual-focus/emotional-entrainment-mechanisms) of the participants in the interaction. Emotional energy is measurable by an index of the attention and involvement produced.

The theory of ritual interaction – like that we endeavour to outline here – is also a theory of situations where shared symbols create long-lasting, or ritually renewed, emotional energy. The dynamics of the ritual, if on the one hand, is associated with the shared symbols, on the other it requires a hoarding of social capital or generalized levels of trust among those who experience the same ritualized situation. It is an emotional substratum (moral density) which legitimizes the social ritual of the proximity violence of a context which justifies its situational frame. If we observe the dynamics that characterize religious rites we can see how they always possess an extremely high degree of social density. It is possible to note that every social system provides formal rituals possessed of an institutional and official profile as well as of natural rituals which arise spontaneously and participate unknowingly to define momentary solidarity and, again, ineffective (or hollow) rituals, unable to produce emotional involvement or group cohesion because of their very unproductivity.

What permits a situation to become a naturally legitimized ritual within a context is when it proves to be unsuitable, and a discrepancy arises between the situation and the context. Therefore, proximity violence delineates a frame defining a ritual, legitimized by a situation and shared at a level of mutually shared temporal experience.

1.7 Proximity Violence Versus Proximity Vulnerability

A woman's body is the "primary place where violence is concretised" (Corradi, 2009: 11). The marriage markets of child brides, outdoor prostitution, or genital mutilation are just some of the aspects of segregationist and patriarchal cultures whose chosen victims are women and girls. Similar practices are an integral part of the established, everyday reality of some migratory cultures, based on VAW as vulnerable subjects.

The term vulnerability/vulnerable comes from the Latin *vulnus* and indicates a wound but also the quality of those who may be injured easily. Vulnerability is primarily a physical condition attributed generally to women exposed to violation of the body. It describes the extreme situation where a person "has no other effective and acceptable choice than to surrender to the abuse of which she is a victim" (art. 4 Directive 36/2011). A woman's body is exposed to this *vulnus* and to the procedural strategies, intimate rituals, relational arrangements defining the exploitation of the vulnerable subject in peculiar situations and contexts. In enduring abuse, the victim is treated not only physically but relationally, that is, she is exposed to the indirect, symbolic violence of the other stemming from the patriarchal culture that legitimizes male power.

Therefore, a woman victim of violence is vulnerable on three fronts (Penedo & Wrabetz, 2015):

1. A pre-existing one, where vulnerability depends, above all, on her background, her family circumstances and the beliefs they imparted, on her physical and psychological condition, her age, and the secondary socialization agents she has had. Non-membership of a social network of individuals who take care of and watch out for each other also determine vulnerability as a pre-existing factor.
2. A contextual one, which reinforces her situational condition of vulnerability. We refer to the legal system and institutions which do not address the marginalizing conditions of social, cultural, or linguistic poverty of the vulnerable subject.
3. A circumstantial one which is created or maintained due to contingent events like unemployment or determined by ensuing factors like illness or accidental events that impact on the existence of certain individuals.

In our opinion, vulnerability is not an intrinsic material characteristic of the human being (Farmer, 2003), but rather a situational trait determined by given contexts and situations. It is a primarily institutional and contextual condition (Fineman, 2015), strongly determined by institutions or a lack of institutions meant to provide the economic, cultural, and social resources which should permit the most fragile subjects to defend themselves. Secondly, vulnerability is situational, that is, it is determined by interpersonal relationships (primary, secondary) which reinforce conditions of vulnerability. Violence in intimate relationships is clearly connected to man's attempt to control and dominate women, and the nature and level of such behaviour varies from culture to culture and appears to be particularly intense in some types of society. "Socio-cultural factors play a significant role in man's possessiveness and connected behaviour" (Dobash & Dobash, 2016: 27). The latter would not be explained, however, if we did not refer to a situational dimension in which it is the victim's vulnerability that does not find escape routes.

This condition of vulnerability is realized within particular contexts of cultural and material poverty but also and above all within relationships of proximity where the oppression of the strongest over more vulnerable subjects is constant. Take one of the many examples of women who lived in deviant family contexts as children, where economic poverty was extreme (situational factor), and cultural and social capital (social ties) was almost non-existent. In all likelihood, these girls were offered two possibilities: in the best of hypotheses, they would marry within the same context of material and moral poverty, based, in any case, on male supremacy subjecting them to a long-lasting "natural life". In the worst-case scenario, they would end up on the streets.

Suppose that if those same women-girls had found opportunities at school, were provided for by social services and institutions which strengthened their precarious condition at cultural and social level, their fate would have changed. This hypothesis is, unfortunately, very far from the reality of the thousands of migrant women who arrive in Europe every year. For these women, the only way to survive is submission as his submissive accomplice to a strong male. When we try to define this (in our opinion) inseparable violence-vulnerability binomial, we need to highlight the complex network of causes that determine the subjugation of a person, since violence not only acts upon but also through bodies, in a blend of complicity, consent, and need for recognition on the part of the victim. As Butler writes, "the very fact of being bound up with others establishes the possibility of being subjugated and exploited" (2000: 61), but each abuse becomes such only under particular circumstances. For all these reasons and the ideas provided so far, it would be better to talk about an inseparable binomial of proximity vulnerability and proximity violence.

The subjugation of the weakest person at emotional level, too, and the consequent self-perception of her vulnerability by the victim, take place within relationships based on the proximity violence perpetrated by the other. He exploits the victim's vulnerability by repeatedly injuring her until the wound is normalized. Violence does not act only on the bodies but also through bodies, in a melange of complicity, consensus, and the need for acknowledgment on the part of the victim. The very fact of being bound to others establishes the possibility of being subjugated and exploited. But it also establishes the possibility of being relieved of suffering, of knowing justice, even love (Butler & Gambetti, 2016).

A wide range of testimonies describes an initial deception perpetrated by the person closest to the victim, who triggers off processes of resilience and individual resistance. Several testimonies describe the victim's difficulty in recognizing the deception and abuse themselves.

Resilience is the victim's internal capability to survive the horror of violence, despite the abuse/mutilations the body has been subjected to. It is a sort of readjustment of the subject. But it alone would not suffice to explain the victim's endurance unless we resort to something else. This allows us to hypothesize the emergence of opaque forms of emotional reluctance. These become a kind of wall of self-defence built by the victim to justify the suffering undergone, sweetening it, making it less unacceptable. This reluctance lies somewhere between the victims' resilience and their capacity for resistance, intended as both compensatory strategies which, if, on the one hand favour the physical subordination of the exploited persons to the will of the trafficker, and on the other permit self-justification of dependence and subordination by the victims. Resistance as a personal interpretation of the violence suffered indicates the victim's unconscious determination not to acknowledge the violence experienced, attributing it to causes of "force majeure". Resistance is a capacity for self-narration of violence in its watered-down form, to make it bearable, and, in some cases, acceptable. Resilience and resistance are meant as compensatory practices which, if, on the one hand justify the subordination of the body of the victim to the will of the perpetrator, on the other provide the victim with self-justification of her dependence and subjection.

Therefore, the victim's will to remain in a condition of subordination cannot be attributed solely to relationships based on dominion and violence. It is a particular form of resistance, activated within a proximity's relationship to make the violence suffered acceptable.

References

Appiah, A. (2010). *The honor code: How moral revolutions happen*. Toronto, ON: Northon and Company.

Arbel, E., Dauvergne, C., & Millbank, J. (2014). *Gender in refugee law: From the margins to the Centre*. London/New York: Routledge.

Bartholini, I. (2013). *Violenza di prossimità. La vittima, il carnefice, lo spettatore e il "grande occhio"*. Milan, Italy: FrancoAngeli.

Bartholini, I. (Ed.). (2015). *Violenza di genere e percorsi mediterranei. Voci, saper, uscite*. Milan, Italy: Guerini e Associati.

Bartholini, I. (2016). Emancipazione pubblica privata. Tratteggi di una gender violence tardo moderna nell'incrociarsi di paradigmi atlantici e mediterranei. *Autonomie locali e servizio sociale, 2*(3), 56–81.

Bartholini, I. (2019). Meticciamento regressivo: donne migranti e donne palermitane. *Sociologia e ricerca sociale, 2*, 29–56.

Bartky, L. S. (1990). *Femininity and domination: Studies in the phenomenology of oppression*. New York: Routledge.

Basaglia, A., Lotti, M., Misiti M., & Tola, V. (2007). *Il silenzio e le parole. II Rapporto nazionale Rete Antiviolenza tra le città Urban-Italia*. Retrieved from: http://www.pariopportunita.provincia.tn.it/filesroot/Documents/approfondimenti/RicercaVilenza_silenzioeparole2009.pdf

Berger, P., & Luckmann, T. (1966). *The social construction of reality*. London: Anchor.

Bernstein, E. (2007). Sex work for the middle classes. *Sexualities, X*(4), 472–488.

Bimbi, F. (2012). *I vocabolari della violenza*. Milan, Italy: Guerrini.

Bimbi, F. (2015). Onore e vergogna. Il ritorno di un paradigma del dibattito europeo. In I. Bartholini (Ed.), *Violenza di genere e percorsi mediterranei* (pp. 27–44). Milan, Italy: Guerini e Associati.

Bimbi, F., & Basaglia, A. (Eds.). (2013). *Speak Out! Migranti e Mentor di comunità contro la violenza di genere*. Padova, Italy: Cleup.

BMBF. (2009). *Tradition and violence against women.* Federal Chancellery Federal Minister for Women and Civil Service Owner. Retrieved from bmbf.gv.at/frauen/migrantinnen/traditionundgewaltanfrauen

Bourdieu, P. (1998). *Male domination.* Paris, France: Galimard.

Bracke, S. (2016). Bouncing back: Vulnerability and resistance in times of resilience. In J. Butler, Z. Gambetti, & L. Sabsay (Eds.), *Vulnerability and resistance* (pp. 52–75). Durham, NC: Duke University Press.

Butler, J. (2000). "https://archive.org/details/antigonesclaim00judi" *Antigone's claim kinship between life and death.* New York: Columbia University.

Butler, J. (2004). *Undoing gender.* Abignton, UK: Routledge.

Butler, J. (2008). Sexual politics, torture, and secular time. *The British Journal of Sociology, 59*(1), 1–23.

Butler, J. (2011). *Creating capabilities. The human development approach.* Cambridge, MA/London: The Belknap Press of Harvard University Press.

Butler, J., & Gambetti, Z. (2016). In L. Sabsay (Ed.), *Vulnerability in resistance.* Durham, NC: Duke University Press.

Casique, L., & Furegato, A. R. F. (2006). Violence against women: Theoretical reflections. *Revista Latino- Americana de Enfermagem, 14*(6), 950–956.

Cassano, F., & Zolo, D. (Eds.). (2007). *L'alternativa mediterranea.* Milan, Italy: Feltrinelli.

Coin, F. (2004). *Gli immigrati, il lavoro, la casa.* Milan, Italy: FrancoAngeli.

Collins, R. (2008). *Violence. A micro-sociological theory.* Princeton, NJ: Princeton University Press.

Connell, R. W. (2002). *Gender.* Cambridge, UK: Polity Press.

Corradi, C. (2005). *Il nemico intimo. Una lettura sociologica dei casi di Novi Ligure e Cogne.* Milan, Italy: Meltemi.

Corradi, C. (2009). *Sociologia della violenza. Identità, modernità, potere.* Rome, Italy: Meltemi.

Corradi, L., & Connell, R. (2014). *Il silenzio della terra. Sociologia Postcoloniale, realtà aborigene e l'importanza del luogo.* Milan, Italy/Udine, Italy: Mimesis.

Council of Europe Convention on preventing and combating violence against women and domestic violence. (2011). Retrieved from: https://www.coe.int/en/web/conventions/full-list/-/conventions/treaty/210

Crenshaw, K. (1991). Mapping the margins: Intersectionality, identity politics, and violence against women of color. *Stanford Law Review, 43*(6), 1241–1299.

Crisp, J., Morris, T., & Refstie, H. (2012). Displacement in urban areas: New challenges, new partnerships. *Disasters, 36*(1), 23–42.

De Beauvoir, S. (1949). *Le Deuxième Sexe.* Paris, France: Gallimard.

Dobash, R., & Dobash, R. (2016). *When men murder women.* New York: Oxford University Press.

Fanon, F. (1961). *Les damnés de la terre.* Paris, France: Maspéro.

Farmer, P. (2003). *Pathologies of power: Health, human rights, and the new war on the poor.* Berkeley, CA: University of California Press.

Fernandez-Alvarez, O. (2014). Non-hegemonic masculinity against gen-der violence. PROCEDIA. *Social and Behavioral Sciences, 161*, 48–55.

Filosof, F. (2000). Violenza economica come contesto alla violenza domestica. In P. Romito (Ed.), *Violenze alle donne e risposte delle istituzioni* (pp. 39–48). Milan, Italy: FrancoAngeli.

Fineman, M. (2008). The vulnerable subject: Anchoring equality in the human condition. *Yale Journal of Law & Feminism, 20*(1), 1–23.

Fineman, M. (2015). *The concept of exploitation in the trafficking in persons protocol.* Vienna, Austria: UNODC.

Foucault, M. (1976). *La Volonté de savoir.* Paris, France: Gallimard.

Friedan, B. (1963). *The feminine mystique.* New York: W.W. Norton Company.

Gagnon, J. H. (2004). *An interpretation of desire.* Chicago: University of Chicago Press.

Garcia-Moreno, C., Jansen, H., Ellsberg, M., Heise, L., & Watts, C. (2006). Prevalence of intimate partner violence: Findings from the WHO multi- multi-country study on women's health and domesticviolence. *Lancet, 368*(9543), 1260–1269.

Gillioz, L., De Puy, J., & Ducret, V. (2000). La violenza domestica in Svizzera: nuovi dati su un fenomeno antico. In P. Romito (Ed.), *Violenze alle donne e risposte delle istituzioni* (pp. 83–96). Milan, Italy: FrancoAngeli.

Giordano, C. (1994). *Der Ehrkomplex im Mittelmeerraum: sozialanthropologische Konstruktion oder Grundstruktur mediterraner Lebensform?* Frankfurt a.M., Germany: Suhrkamp Verlag.

Goffman, E. (1974). *Frame analysis: An essay on the organization of experience*. New York: Harper &Row.

Goffman, E. (1976). *Gender advertisements*. Cambridge, UK: Harvard University Press.

Gracia, E., & Lila, M. (2015). *Attitudes towards violence against women in the EU*. European Commission. DG JUST. Retrieved from: https://publications.europa.eu/en/publication-detail/-/publication/a8bad59d-933e-11e5-983e-01aa75ed71a1/language-en

Hakim, C. (2015). Economies of desire: Sexuality and the sex industry in the twenty-first century. *Economic Affairs, 35*(3), 329–348.

Haraway, D. (1988). Situated knowledges: The science question in feminism and the privilege of partial perspective. *Feminist Studies, 14*(3), 575–599.

Herzfeld, M. (1980). Honour and shame: Problems in the comparative analysis of moral systems. *Man, 16*, 339–351.

Illouz, E. (2007). *Cold intimacies: The making of emotional capitalism*. Cambridge, UK: Polity Press.

Irigaray, L. (1992). *Io, tu, Noi. Per una cultura della differenza*. Turin, Italy: Bollati Boringhieri.

Istanbul Convention (2011). Council of Europe Convention on preventing and combating violence against women and domestic violence, Council of Europe Treaty Series No. 210 (https://rm.coe.int/168008482e)

Jaji, R. (2009). Masculinity on unstable ground: Young refugee men in Nairobi. *Journal of Refugee Studies, 22*(2), 177–194.

Kapur, R. (2002). The tragedy of victimization rhetoric: Resurrecting the "native" subject in international/post-colonial feminist legal politics. *Harvard Human Rights Journal, 15*(1), 1–38.

Kirby, P. (2006). *Vulnerability and violence: The impact of globalization*. London: Pluto Press.

Krause-Vilmar, J. (2011). *Preventing gender-based violence: Building livelihoods. Guidance and tools for improved programming, women's refugee commission*. Retrieved from: https://reliefweb.int/report/world/toolkit-optimizing-cash-based-interventions-protection-gender-based-violence.

Lerner, G. (1986). *The creation of patriarchy*. New York/Oxford, UK: Oxford University Press.

Mackenzie, C., Rogers, W., & Dodds, S. (2014). *Vulnerability: New essays in ethics and Femminist philosophy*. Oxford, UK: Oxford University Press.

MacKinnon, C. A. (1989). *Toward a feminist theory of the state*. Cambridge, UK: Harvard University Press.

Mackinnon, C. A. (2006). *Are women human?* Cambridge, UK: Harvard University Press.

Manifesto REds.tockings. (1969). Retrieved from: https://archive.org/stream/REds.tockingsManifesto/REds.tockings-Manifesto_djvu.txt

Merry, S. E. (2009). *Gender violence: A cultural perspective*. Chichester, UK: Wiley-Blackwell.

Mitchell, J. (1984). *Women, the longest revolution*. New York: Pantheon Books.

Morgan, K., & Thapar-Björkert, S. (2006a). I'd rather you'd lay me on the floor and start kicking me: Understanding symbolic violence in everyday life. *Women's Studies International Forum, 29*, 441–452.

Morgan, K., & Thapar-Björkert, S. (2006b). "I'd rather you'd lay me on the floor and start kicking me": Understanding symbolic violence in everyday life. *Women's Studies International Forum, 29*(5), 489–498.

Moscovici, S. (1984). The phenomenon of social representations. In S. Moscovici & R. Farr (Eds.), *Social representations*. Cambridge, UK: Cambridge University Press.

Nagguja, et al. (2014). *From the frying pan to the fire. Psychosocial challenges faced by vulnerable refugee women and girls in Kampala*. Kampala, Uganda: Refugee Law Project.

Nussbaum, M. (2000). *Women and human development: The capabilities approach*. Cambridge: University Press.

Nussbaum, M. (2011). *Creating capabilities: The human development approach*. Cambridge, MA: The Belknap Press of Harvard University Press.

Peano, I. (2013). Opaque loves: Governance and escape in the intimate sphere of Nigerian sex workers. *Etnografia e Ricerca Qualitativa, 3*, 359–384.

Penedo, R., & Wrabetz, J. (2015). Trafficking in human beings in time and space. A socioecological perspective. In M. J. Guia (Ed.), *The illegal business of human trafficking* (pp. 1–19). Cham, Switzerland: Springer Nature Switzerland.

Peristiany, J. (1965). *Honor and shame: The values of Mediterranean society*. London: Weidenfeld & Nicolson.

Phillips, A. (2013). *Our bodies, whose property?* Princeton, NJ: Princeton University Press.

Pinelli, B. (2011). Attraversando il mediterraneo. Il "Sistema campo" in Italia: violenza e soggettività nelle esperienze delle donne. *Lares, 77*(1), 159–179.

Preciado, P. B. (2014). *Pornotopia: An essay on Playboy's architecture and biopolitics*. New York: Zone Books.

Råheim, M., Magnussen, L., Sekse, R., Lunde, A., Jacobsen, T., & Blystad, A. (2016). Researcher–researched relationship in qualitative research: Shifts in positions and researcher vulnerability. *International Journal Qualitative Studies Health Well-being, 11*. Retrieved from: https://www.ncbi.nlm.nih.gov/pmc/articles/PMC4910304/

Razack, S., Smith, M., & Thobani, M. (Eds.). (2011). *States and races. Critical Femminist for the 21st century*. Toronto, ON: Between the Lines.

Romito, P. (2000). *La violenza di genere su donne e minori*. Milan, Italy: FrancoAngeli.

Rubin, A. (1997). Conflict and continuity. *Journal of Communication, 47*(4), 4–5.

Said, E. (1993). *Culture and imperialism*. London: Chatto & Windus.

Schütz, A. (1956). *Der sinnhafte Aufbau der sozialen Welt. Eine Einleitung in die Verstehende Soziologie*. Frankfurt a.M., Germany: Suhrkamp Verlag.

Siegel, J. P. (2013). Breaking the links in intergenerational violence: An emotional regulation perspective. *Family Process, 52*(2), 163–178.

Tajfel, H. (1981). *Human groups and social categories*. Cambridge, UK: Cambridge University Press.

Tognetti, M., & Rossi, P. (Eds.). (2016). *Salute e inclusione sociale degli immigrati. La sfida dell'accesso ai servizi sanitari*. Milan, Italy: FrancoAngeli.

Turnaturi, G. (2012). *Vergogna. Metamorfosi di un'emozione*. Rome, Italy: Feltrinelli.

Volpato, C. (2011). *Deumanizzazione. Come si legittima la violenza*. Rome, Italy/Bari, Italy: Laterza.

Volpato, C. (2013). *Psicosociologia del maschilismo*. Rome, Italy/Bari, Italy: Laterza.

Walby, S. (1990). *Theorizing patriarchy*. Cambridge, UK: Basic Blackwell.

WHO. (2002). *Violenza e la salute nel mondo. Rapporto dell'organizzazione mondiale della sanità, Quaderni di sanità pubblica*, CIS Ed.e, Milan. Retrieved from: https://apps.who.int/iris/bitstream/handle/10665/42495/9241545615_ita.pdf;jsessionid=C9F6C63C30A159DE33E6BBDE85C323F9?sequence=5

WHO. (2005). *Multi country study on women's health and domestic violence against women*. Geneva, Switzerland: WHO Press.

Wiederman, M. W. (2000). Women's body image self-consciousness during physical intimacy with a partner. *Journal of Sex Research, 36*, 60–68.

Chapter 2
Deception and Abuse: Manifold Instances of Proximity Violence Against Sub-Saharan Women

2.1 Introduction

The extreme variety of migrant women's experiences is reflected in the diversity of the situations in which they undergo discrimination and violence. What appears, however, to be explored to a lesser degree are the mechanisms that make it possible to continue a violent relationship, whereby categories like "gender", "power", and "domain" may prove insufficient. The Recommendations and Conventions that have been drafted at the international and European level, and which have subsequently informed national legislation, fail to free themselves from this impasse.

1. General Recommendation n.19, 11th session of the United Nations, art. 1 establishes, incontrovertibly, that VAW is a form of "gender-based" discrimination and "as that violence directed against a person based on his/her gender. It includes acts that inflict physical, mental or sexual harm or suffering, threats of such acts, coercion and other deprivations of liberty".
2. The Council of Europe Convention on Preventing and Combating Violence (*Istanbul Convention*) defines gender violence, as "any violence directed against a woman as such, or affecting women disproportionately" (Article 3).

The violence experienced by more vulnerable subjects during migration throws considerable light on the comprehension of the mechanisms permitting it to express itself, explain its genesis and development, its normalization, its reproduction and representation. Gender relations in areas of the Mediterranean cannot be interpreted by means of a single currently acknowledged paradigm, but are themselves the product of a hybrid cluster of diverse cultural influences. The Mediterranean is, today, a crucible, where uninterrupted behavioural patterns favouring interweaves of violent conduct, legitimated by sexist logic and patriarchal reverberations, persist. (Bartholini, 2016; Edwards, 1987; Garcia-Moreno, Jansen, Ellsberg, Heise, & Watts, 2006).

I. Bartholini, *The Trap of Proximity Violence*,
https://doi.org/10.1007/978-3-030-52451-7_2

The most recent migratory arrivals have also contributed to the re-emergence of the "honour-and-shame" paradigm (Giordano, 1994; Peristiany, 1965), "expressed primarily through gender-oriented relations founded on control of women" (Bimbi, 2015: 22) within marital and parental relationships. As Bimbi wrote recently, "the honour-and-shame paradigm is a characteristic of the Mediterranean area" (ibidem: 46); even if it seems to represent an archaic residue, it continues to be rampant amid groups of newcomers, also in terms of manifest violence.

One of the most devastating effects of this paradigm is legitimization of the sexual exploitation of migrants from Africa (especially Nigeria). Furthermore, it also emphasizes forms of gender submission found within more traditional marriage-based relationships. The issue of female subordination and exploitation may, therefore, be attributed to the cultural models underlying the socialization processes experienced by migrant women in their native lands and reproduced in their host countries. From this angle, violence can act as a social force – endowed, therefore, with the ability to structure reality (Corradi, 2009). The logical, consequential assumption is that there is almost always a continuum between situations of domination and exploitation and the perpetration of violent acts against women (Collins, 2008; Corradi & Stöckl, 2016; Filosof, 2000; Gillioz, De Puy, & Ducret, 2000; Reale, 2000; Romito, 2000).

To consider violence as belonging to the "normality" of relationships marked by female submission and, in extreme cases, by outdoor prostitution, becomes sociologically useful to in-depth studies of processes and representations which contribute to the perpetuation of male power within the realm of gender relations, even among social groups that may be identified directly with the marginality or deviance found in some migratory contexts. The more representations legitimizing the centuries-old exercise of control by men over women's bodies are shared socially, the more they relegate women to positions of subjugation and vulnerability.

In this chapter the author analyses some of the role positions emerging from the gender dynamics found among migrants, shedding light on possible processes of submission and internalization of mechanisms of gender subalternity in the countries where migrants arrive and on the viscous links between vulnerability and resistance characterizing women victims who have experienced various kinds of proximity violence. She also foregrounds some of the equivocations surrounding affective action declined in feminine terms and instrumental action declined in masculine terms (Bracke, 2016), suggesting that the proximity variety may be considered a more "intimate and deceptive" form of gender violence.

2.2 Mechanisms of Proximity Violence

Traditionally, violence involves forms of social exclusion, discrimination (Jaji, 2009), secondary victimization (Pinelli, 2011), exploitation of labour (Coin, 2004), forced prostitution (Krause-Vilmar, 2011), and sexual abuse (Crisp, Morris, & Refstie, 2012). Although recent literature has defined gender-based violence broadly as the exercise of physical and psychological dominion over the victim, highlighted the various modalities (direct, indirect, physical, symbolic, cultural, instrumental, etc.) that explicitly explain it, the issue remains within a cultural paradigm which tolerates, when it does not actually legitimate, gender inequality. Gender differences are the basis of male domination over (Bourdieu, 1998) and the abuse of women.

In the following pages, we argue that a certain kind of violence is not "violence against women" or "gender-based violence", but is a specific, distinct type of violence belonging to the realm of proximity relationships, and which we may well define as the violence of proximity. In similar relationships, the perpetrator is not a "neutral subject", but the person most intimate and closest to the victim at an emotional and life-plan level.

The acts of violence immigrant women and refugees/asylum seekers are faced with are often linked to the genealogy and intimacy legitimizing – by virtue of parental or emotional ties – the exercise of patriarchal power over them. At other times, the violence undergone bears testimony to marriage agreements, sometimes to sex-trade pacts where the victims are passively vulnerable. The symbolic device making all of this possible is that whereby parental or parental-based authority provides traffickers with the sceptre of power over women and their bodies.

What we notice is that relationships involving proximity violence dehumanize the victim's physical dimension while also justifying the abuse perpetrated by virtue of aspects that can be ascribed to a traditional act or to a joint affective and traditional act. Those who use violence exploiting the body of the other for sexual, procreative, commercial purposes and, at the same time, make use of them as tools of higher, affective or moral, order.

Recognizing the violence of proximity in migrants who flock to reception centres or walk the city streets often poses interpretative and operational difficulties to reception-centre caretakers when fighting abuse and taking charge of victims (Bartholini, 2020). In gender relations it is the symbolic and material oppression, culturally normalized and internalized by victims, which makes them acquiescent and often "collaborative" with respect to the "proximate" perpetrator. This is due to their own vulnerability, but also to their sentimental and/or fiduciary dependence, which becomes resistance, adaptation to certain situations and their own condition.

Upon an emotional plane, we find the dynamics of trust, sentimental closeness, or psychological oppression that determine acceptance of violence by the victim. The hope of a better future is used as a lever by the perpetrator to coerce the victim to accept the squalor of the present as a necessary part of the plan for improvement. The violence suffered by the victim is itself the fruit of resistance against putting an end to the relationship with the perpetrator.

The *proximus* is the other who, in a rapport of physical and spatial proximity, occupies a dominant position. As this dominance is almost always explicitly founded on gender difference, on direct and indirect physical and psychological abuse of the victim, perpetrated in a temporal *dureé*, it may be deemed to belong to the category of proximity. The category of proximity, which illuminates the intimate character of the relationship, makes violence within the victim–perpetrator dyad and the exploitation of the victim outside the relationship too (as in the case of sexual exploitation) possible. Gender itself may, therefore, be considered "a fluctuating artifice, an incessant work in progress, a practice of improvisation within a scenario of constraint, which does not recuse violence but presupposes it" (Butler, 2004: 26) within a mechanism of proximity. Gender is a variable favouring proximity violence which, however, does not justify it completely.

As far as the victim is concerned, the perpetrator is in an asymmetrical, prevaricating position. From this point of view, the possibility of carrying out violence is subordinate to the behaviour of the perpetrator who dominates the victim who finds herself in a condition of absolute vulnerability due to the situation. However, the persistence of the victim within a condition of subordination cannot be attributed solely to relationships based on dominion, but rather to action grounded in affection, emotion, or trust, which make the victim docile towards or accepting of violence.

Contrary to all supposition, the victim's humanity is recognized by the perpetrator. Dehumanizing the other is a practice that allows you to inhibit feelings that we attribute to a human being. The violence of proximity does not dehumanize the victim but places herself in an alliance with his perpetrator, and makes her feel she is an active part of the relationship. Proximity violence is multifaceted, is always and in any case legitimized so that it triggers mechanisms of resistance within the victim. It adapts to people and relationships, and, from time to time, takes forms that the victim can still bear. The victim adheres to the role assigned, makes it her own because she is involved in a situation where the context provides no glimmer of the change. In other words, it renders the victim resistant within the dynamics of proximity violence.

The example of the women, victims of gender and/or sexual exploitation, interviewed here, seems to confirm this hypothesis.

Proximity violence is a particularly substantial risk for the majority of migrants, precisely because exogenous and endogenous factors of their lives intersect. These do not concern the asymmetry of power alone but the social ambit within which it is structured. In the case of migrant women, we find three variables: their material living conditions which make them vulnerable in terms of daily life; their subjective condition which makes some of them particularly susceptible to violence; situations of temporary difficulty which gradually arise to aggravate already precarious conditions. The persistence, however, of the vulnerable subject within dynamics of subordination (Kirby, 2006), cannot be attributed solely to relationships based on domination, but rather to the viscosity of mechanisms based on dependence and a strong tendency to resist within vulnerability, which render the victim docile and inclined to normalize violence even in the presence of possible ways out. The "fatal" mix lies in the intertwining of vulnerability and resistance. As Butler writes, "we cannot understand bodily vulnerability outside [...] social and material relations" (2016: 16). Violence takes advantage of intimate spaces, causing deep harm which creates resistance against its own acknowledgement. Evidence of this is that operators struggle to recognize, within the tangled skein of the needs migrant women bear, exposure to violence if not as a secondary phenomenon to a more general dependence that makes the victim's body itself an agency of relationships rather than a material entity.

In fact, "if we also say that the vulnerability to dispossession, poverty, insecurity, and harm that constitutes a precarious position in the world itself leads to resistance, then it seems we reverse the sequence: we are first vulnerable and then overcome that vulnerability, at least provisionally, trough acts of resistance" (ibidem: 12). In other words, the multifactorial vulnerability makes the victim resistant in the dynamics of proximity violence, but also makes it deliberately exposed to the domain of others "an embodied enactment" (ibidem: 22). Violence favours intimacy, causing deep hurt that translates into resistance to recognition of the violence and injury. The proof is that the operators themselves are struggling to recognize, in the tangle of needs with which migrant women are bearers, exposure to violence if not as a secondary phenomenon to a more general dependence that makes the victim's body itself an agency of relationships rather than a material entity.

2.3 From Patriarchy to Proximity Domination

The view that violence is associated with gender as the sphere of a power relationship has become a classic; it is believed to operate in two directions: men's oppression of women through hierarchization of difference (Bourdieu, 1998; Edwards, 1987; Garcia-Moreno et al., 2006); the creation of strict barriers between gender identities (Bimbi, 2015; Butler, 2016; Connell, 2002; Heller, 1985; Nussbaum, 2000). In this sense, gender may be considered "a floating artifice, an incessant work in progress, a practice of improvisation in a scenario of constraint, which does not reject violence but presupposes it" (Butler, 2004: 26) within a mechanism of proximity.

The honour-shame dyad generally typifies pre-modern or archaic societies based on a "bond of reason and emotion, the invention of an enemy to defend the boundaries and rigid identities of a group, the victim's body transformed into the material to be modelled, the spectacular diffusion of the atrocities in the media, the disappearance of the aggressor in a project that dominates it and, together, its protagonism" (Corradi, 2009: 104). In similar cultures, a body is subject to violence insofar as it is the harbinger of shame and dishonour. Since shame constitutes the negative counterpart of honour, it is closely rooted in the way in which different patriarchal cultures interpret and evaluate honour (Heller, 1985; Herzfeld, 1980).

Gender segregation, and the historically acknowledged asymmetry between femininity and masculinity, as defining axes positioned culturally in space and time, lie at the basis of practices aimed at violating women, especially when they are in conditions of vulnerability and not members of a parental circle. The paradigm of male dominion itself (Bourdieu, 1998) and paradigm of patriarchy, indicated "as a system of social structures and practices in which men dominate, oppress and exploit women" (Walby, 1990), are a fundamental lens for understanding the segregationist practices of which migrant women are victims in their countries of origin which contribute in some ways to the exoticization of damaging practices, while "our" western forms of violence against women are considered residues of social pathologies that we are overcoming. The phenomena of marriage markets, child brides, outdoor prostitution of Nigerian women (Peano, 2013; Siegel & De Roos, 2016), as well as genital mutilation also represent some of the aspects of a segregationist and patriarchal type of culture. The risk, however, is that they may be assimilated within the migratory culture of the countries of origin and destination and thus place the vulnerability and resistance of victims "other than us" upon the same level, without evaluating what they suggest and the possible *mestizament* they may have undergone within the contexts of places of departure and arrival.

Reading violence in the "normality" of relationships marked by female subordination within "exotic" contexts, other than tour own, proves sociologically useful when seeking to investigate in-depth representations and dynamics which contribute to the perpetuation of male power within inter-gender relationships (Collins, 2008; Corradi, 2009; Gillioz et al., 2000; Romito, 2000), even in social groups not directly identifiable as migratory areas of marginality or deviance. It becomes especially useful to trace the recurring pattern, "the social order functioning as an immense symbolic machine aimed at ratifying the male domination on which it is based" (Bourdieu, 1998: 15).

By means of traditional rituals or commercial exchange aimed at sexual exploitation, the right of the male over the female body is acknowledged by an agreement between male contractors, one of whom delivers the victim's body to the other party who is then entitled to rape, subjugate, and exploit it. Those who have dominion over the body of others maintain and confirm honour by managing the other by implementing multiple modalities of segregation and abuse. The relationships to which immigrant women and refugees/asylum seekers are subjected often associated genealogy with intimacy and confirm sales agreements, regarding marriage or prostitution, render the victim passively vulnerable. The symbolic device that facilitates all this is the delivery of victims to a blood relation (in some cases, even delivery to a trafficker) authorized to control them. In addition to being characterized by asymmetrical relationships, intra-community hierarchies often base their premises on forms of genealogical calculation (Povinelli, 2002). Besides, honour often constitutes one of the main if not the main factor justifying recourse to violence, after the victim attempts to test or challenge male honour which is measured on the basis of a woman's degree of submission; it is not by the performative effects of the will of the ruler, but in the obedience of the victim that the logic of domination is gauged.

When pinpointing the mechanisms that permit the perpetuation of violent relationships, the categories of "gender", "power", and "dominion", widely represented in the *Convention* and in the *Recommendations*, are aetiologically insufficient. The ways gender-based violence is experienced by migrant women, at both symbolic and actual concrete level, provides proximal relationships with a starting point from which to normalize and reproduce themselves.

To highlight some of the links between the segregationist and pre-modern logics of which the newcomers are bearers, we chose a proximal declination of violence which includes the victim's "resistance" (Butler, 2016) as a factor necessary to its perpetuation. In the following pages, we shall emphasize how this type of violence as a particular form of violence made possible only because of the closeness between perpetrator and victim. In this kind of relationship, the perpetrator is not a "neutral subject", but "the" person or "one" of the people legitimized by patriarchal codes to subject women to their power. In proximity violence it is the symbolic and material oppression by a "neighbour" which renders the victim acquiescent. This is not only due, to some extent, to the vulnerability of the victim but also to her sentimental and/or fiduciary dependence on the perpetrator, which is then transformed into resistance, adaptation to the situation and to the contingent state of affairs.

Proximity violence circumscribes the exploitation and abuse of the victim making her resistant by virtue of its "proximal" characteristics. The perpetrator may be a husband, a partner, a boyfriend even simply a friend in whom the abused person places particular trust. Proximity does not characterize exclusively this type of relationship, but makes violence within the abusive-abused dyad possible, and favours the exploitation of the victim outside the relationship (as in the case of sexual exploitation) in other human settings ordained by the perpetrator himself. That proximus is in a relationship of physical proximity, but particularly occupies a dominant position on the victim's perceptive horizon. Since this predominance is almost always explicitly based on direct and indirect physical and psychological, abuse of the victim, perpetrated over a period of time indicated as *durée*, it may be considered as belonging to the category of proximity. In other words, proximity violence is legitimized by trust and not even by the emotional attachment of the victim in that interpersonal situation and in a context that is arranged according to a patriarchal order.

2.4 Research Carried Out Among Migrant Women Hosted in Shelters and in the *Ballarò* Neighbourhood

2.4.1 Marginal Notes on the Research "Method"

Often, a goodly knowledge of their respondents' backgrounds can help researchers maintain a neutral approach and avoid potential "pollution" of the object of their study. This theoretical approach can prove particularly advantageous when it comes to exploring the behaviour and the interactive dynamics (De Wal, 1992) of human beings (Mason, 2002; Schütz, 1967) and help avoid a priori emphases capable of jeopardizing the results of research at various levels.

The qualitative methodological approach employed in this research, which avails itself of the participant observation method, permitted greater interaction between the researcher and the immigrant women, and had the merit of bringing to the fore answers to invisible questions (Bonner & Tolhurst, 2002; Råheim et al., 2016) while also counting on the contribution of intermediaries who facilitated direct, though temporary, contact with the interviewees (Gorman, Clayton, Shep, & Clayton, 2005).

The fundamental aim of the interviews carried out subsequently as a technique typical of qualitative analysis was not to limit it to the mere collection of information, but consisted in gaining access to the "perspective of the subjects being studied" (Corbetta, 2015: 70), that is, interpretations of their perceptions, feelings or representations of the world as well as of the motivations intrinsic to their actions.

The research carried out between 2016 and 2017 aimed at appraising perceptions of the violence to which sub-Saharan women hosted by various immigrant facilities in Sicily were submitted. Both the migrant women who have lived there for the longest time, and the women who hosted by the SPRAR[1] in the same neighbourhood, belong to family systems free to manage their own daily lives and personal choices.

It was adopted an intersectional approach (Crenshaw, 1991) to analyse the multiple forms of discrimination produced by the specific positions of the interviewees while, at the same time, it sought to detect similarities and differences between the various processes of acknowledgement undertaken. Given the differences between the interviewees – from the Nigerian prostitute to the mother of traditional Islamic faith – the adoption of an intersectional approach, based on the age, education, and class of the interviewees, seemed the most appropriate choice to use to detect the forms of multiple discrimination caused by the interviewees' specific positions and, at the same time, investigate the differences and similarities in the processes of acknowledgement initiated by the interviewees themselves. This approach aimed at considering, simultaneously, all the axes of the subordination experienced by the women while emphasizing the need to distinguish between their cases (Bograd, 1999; Johnson, 2006; Menjìavar & Salcido, 2002; Nixon & Humphreys, 2010) and at considering the vulnerability of which they were carriers as the ante-room of the violence of which they had been victims.

A non-directive interview was outlined and employed with a view to facilitate the interviewees' narratives. The presence of cultural mediators was vital when seeking to grasp the cultural, relational, family backgrounds of the women interviewed, as well as their recollections of the violent experiences and traumas to which they had been subjected, as well as their degrees of awareness of the violence undergone. The interview was divided into 5 thematic areas. The first concerned the women's personal, family, and sentimental backgrounds; the second referred to the physical violence they had experienced, which was usually the first form of violence acknowledged; the third regarded symbolic violence (Bourdieu, 1998), the cultural devices used to legitimize processes of family socialization and naturalization of gender differentiation; the fourth area regarded the process of acknowledgement (or not) of the violence suffered. It was precisely the formulation of a number of specific questions concerning this last-mentioned area which permitted us to comprehend the ways by which normalization of violence within "affective-emotional" contexts of subordination and normalized suffering was achieved. Some short accounts of the most significant testimonies regarding this fourth area are provided below.

---

[1] SPRAR is an acronym for the System for Asylum Seekers and Refugees. It was established in 2002 following a 2001 "protocol", stipulated between the Ministry of Interior, ANCI, and UNHCR. While the CAS are extraordinary reception centers for asylum seekers, the SPRAR is composed of a network of structures, consisting of apartments for a few people up to medium and large structures that welcome different profiles of subjects – by those who have made a request of asylum and comes from a CAS, or is already a beneficiary of some protection or is still a vulnerable person.

Recognizing and hosting refugee—-asylum seekers who are victims of violence, both in their places of origin and during the journey to the European States bordering the Mediterranean, is a problem which raises many questions regarding the situations and conditions regarding reception, and the dynamics of communication and understanding between hosting operators and asylum seekers in order to detect the violence of which asylum seekers are often victims beginning with their own families (Kapur, 2002; Macioti & Pugliese, 2010). The presence of cultural mediators, in the case of the immigrant guests of the SPRARS, of particular stakeholders like teachers of the children of those residing in the *Ballarò* district of Palermo, or of the social workers who regularly meet them, was essential in order to grasp the cultural, family, and relational frameworks of the interviewees themselves and, above all, to spark their memory concerning the violent experiences and the traumas undergone.

The mediators permitted us to assess the degree of awareness of the migrants when it came to the violence they had been subjected to, but also and above all the level of their unawareness often combined with their individual resistance. The narrative, prompted by sporadic questions and directed above all to hearing just how freely the interlocutor wished to communicate, favoured a reinterpretation of the past which led, only in the cases reported below by Aziza, Ghana, and Foluke and, to a sort of re-appropriation of parts of their own life stories to which they were able to restore some accompanied by the intention of achieving a more satisfying life. The interview was divided, therefore, into 4 thematic areas. The first concerned the personal, family, and sentimental aspects of the lives of the women interviewed; the second referred to the physical violence suffered, which was usually the first form of violence they acknowledged; the third regarded symbolic violence and the cultural devices that legitimize it by means of processes of family socialization and the naturalization of gender differentiation; the fourth referred to the pathway taken to acknowledge (or not) the violence suffered and to the resistance processes activated.

It was precisely the formulation of a small number of prompt questions relating to the latter thematic area that permitted us to trace and understand the processes favouring the normalization of violence in an "affective-emotional" context of segregation and patriarchy. The interest of the interviewers did not focus on the experiences of the interviewees, but on the interpretative methods used to process the events, based on the same existential vulnerability that made them resistant as subjects through their own agency and by means of a peculiar world view generated by their own experiences. Below are some of the most significant testimonies relating to the fourth area, which were subsequently divided into main, accessory, and mirror nodes, in order to reconstruct the dynamics of resistance and resilience forming the background and, in the case of mirror nodes, the perceptions and interpretations provided by the Palermitan women living in the same neighbourhood as the migrant women regarding their behaviour and conduct.

The language of the interviewees underwent, even with the help of the mediators, an overall paraphrase as close as possible to the contents, expressed in French or English, even in the dialects of their regions and tribes or through a use, however wavering, of standard Italian or the Sicilian dialect.

The general prompt questions invited the interviewees to tell how they had arrived in Italy; what they had expected to change in their lives after their arrival; what they had done inside the shelters that hosted them or how they lived in the neighbourhood (who they frequented, how they spent their time, etc.) and, above all, how the dynamics of their proximal relationships unfolded, what they remembered best, and what, on the other hand, were unable to forget. The answers given to the same prompts were defined and attributed to the fourth area concerning their pathway to acknowledgement (or not) of the violence undergone and the processes of resistance activated.

The non-directive interviews were the outcome of a lengthy ongoing process used to structure the interview in order to detect and select some sensitizing concepts within the areas of the interview.

During the phase during which the thematic areas were defined, during the experiential stage of the management and production of the nodes, and, lastly, during that of the coding and interpretation of the material gathered, "the interview was always seen as complex social interaction" (Ferrarotti, 1989: 26), where the construction and attribution of meaning concerning the experiences narrated foresaw mutual trust.

The administration of the interviews was followed by a phase where the transcripts were read and reread as were the "memos", the short notes written by the interviewers during the interviews, and which regarded, mostly, observations of the interviewees' behaviour, particular posture, tone of voice, pauses, or digressions.

The material collected and examined was then divided into sensitizing nodes or concepts (Blumer, 1969), corresponding to the non-directive interview's conceptual categories and those of the focus groups previously identified, using the NVivo 12 software (Non-numerical Unstructured Data Indexing, Searching and Theorizing Vivo).

The peculiarity of the NVivo software is that it fosters the collection of unstructured data belonging to the same procedural scheme, acting as a sort of hypertext. While imposing an orderly system on the researcher, besides on a *Document System*, it rests on a system of containers – called (main) nodes or categories – which serve to handle coding, i.e. the attribution of segment codes of text to the interview material. NVivo was used during both the conceptualization and the creative phases by identifying and examining accessory nodes, in order to provide a more analytical visualization of the coded texts. It contributed to the examination of the attributes, to view the documents with which a specific value was associated. Finally, it permitted the identification of "hybrid" textual passages within a node. The three operations also favoured the enhancement of secondary elements of the interviews which were associated with broader and more distinguishable textual material in the four main interview categories.

For these characteristics, it was deemed beneficial to use the NVivo software for a more in-depth analysis of the fourth category.

The result was a complex network of:

1. main nodes, or emerging categories, identified in the testimonies of Ghana, Foluke, and Aziza,

2. accessory nodes, describing experiences which we believed supported the three main categories and which recurred in most of the interviews conducted with the migrants.

Main nodes

	Abuse	deception	sexual violence
1st accessory node ***role subordination,***	2nd accessory node ***economic dependence,***	3rd accessory node ***motherhood, decided by the partner***	4th accessory node ***uncritical acceptance of past models***

In this chapter, two parts of the material deriving from the interviews corresponding to the main issues are reported below: abuse, described by Ghana; deception, testified by Foluke; the violence of a forced marriage, as told by Aziza.

2.4.2 *Ghana, Foluke, and Aziza*

2.4.2.1 Ghana and Her Abuse-Ridden Journey

Ghana began by describing the hopes she had nourished before boarding the boat she took. She meant to arrive in Italy and find a job to help her family which was in economic difficulty. Once on board, two men approached her asking if she knew how to make love with a man or whether she was a virgin. At this point the interviewee said that.

Despite not wishing to answer two strange men regarding this overly intimate sphere of my life, I could not but answer and that is how my long journey of pain, hatred and despair began.

The girl spoke very softly, her gaze fixed on the floor, as she told of how she had been raped repeatedly by these two men, whose physiognomies she could not remember, because she had never found the courage to look them in the face. They kept telling her that only constant training would prepare her for the employment awaiting her in Italy.

2.4.2.2 Foluke and a Post-journey Scam

Foluke arrived in Italy, like many other women, in hopes of enjoying a better life style. In reality, she had been tricked by a female friend, because, once she landed in Sicily, she was obliged to become a prostitute. During her paid sexual work, she established a "sentimental" rapport with one of her clients, Michele, with whom she also had a child. Despite going to live together, Michele made her continue to work as a prostitute because he had no intention of having a child, much less pay for its upkeep. Furthermore, as Michele was unemployed, he kept telling Foluke that "she had to manage things herself!"

So, I continued prostituting myself, and with the little money made, I needed mainly to satisfy the needs of Michele who smoked, went to the bar and always liked to have new clothes to cut a good figure. What was left was for my son; for me there was not even a euro.

2.4.2.3 Aziza and the Domestic Violence of a Forced Marriage

The case of Aziza, a woman from Cameroon, is emblematic. At 14 years she was obliged by her own family to marry a man of 35.

This is her story:

> *I had no idea what was happening to me. I found myself in the home of an unknown man whom I had married at my father's behest. I had to look after him, cook ... but worst thing of all ...the word ugly does not suffice ... I'm looking for a stronger one ... the most animalistic thing he did ... was that he took me to bed continuously against my will. As soon as he came home, I shuddered, because whatever I was doing, I had to stop and give myself to him against my will. I could not refuse him. I could not turn back. I don't want to remember; it makes me suffer and I still feel great pain when I think about it.*

For Aziza, like the majority of the interviewees, violence was a necessary rite of passage in their life stories.

Male hegemony was considered normal by most of the interviewees, as were the non-negotiable rules of family life. Only the violence undergone during their journeys towards the shores of the Mediterranean was considered "abnormal" though necessary for their very survival. In these cases, the abnormality did not reside in the act as such, but in identifying the actor as an outsider, not an insider, in terms of family relationships. Some of the women told about the ways in which they had been tricked into leaving their own countries only to find themselves entangled in a skein of forced prostitution. For some of the interviewees, prostitution was perceived as a "necessary evil", an inevitable, mandatory condition to be spoken about only sotto voce, however. These women's stories also caused the "racialization of identities and violence as culture-specific" (Hajdukowski-Ahmed, Khanlou, & Moussa, 2009: 6). At the same time, the tendency of considering the women as incapable to survive within the foreign environments and even to adapt to new situations in the countries of resettlement makes their perpetrator s stronger.

From the non-directive interviews conducted, it is evident that the practice implemented within a patriarchal culture, involved continuous "testing" of an "intimate contract" between victim and perpetrator, is confirmed by the passive resistance manifested by the victim, and her consequent, continuous renewal of consent involving the hetero-management of her existence. Here, resistance means being consciously exposed to power and the need to face its most deleterious effects without, however, releasing oneself from dependence. From this angle, the resistance of a vulnerable subject does favour possible emancipation from the condition of exposure to the power of the other, but underpins the victim's permanence in the condition in which she has come to find herself (Butler, 2004, 2016). The reiteration of the violence suffered is itself a consequence of the victim's resistance against severing the dynamic ties that make her a victim of her perpetrator. Male domination, and the way in which it is not only imposed but undergone, is the consequence of resistance on the part of the victim, used to avoid a condition/situation that she does not fully recognize in all its gravity, precisely because of the oppressive and sentimental/fiduciary relationship that binds her to her perpetrator. In other cases, it is the hope of a better future that is used as a lever by the perpetrator to force the victim to accept a present where she is subjected to deception and sexual exploitation as a necessary part of a plan to improve her condition. From this point of view, Illouz (2008) and Bernstein (2007) have amply highlighted the progressive penetration of commercial logic into sexual relations. This logic is acceptable to the victim only within the dynamics where responsibility for ownership of the female body due to patriarchal cultures as well as emotional dependence acts as a cement between the victim and her perpetrator.

2.4.3 Accessory Nodes: Evidence of Female Subordination and the "Perfect" Marriage

The three women, from different parts of Africa, who arrived in Italy through the Libyan-Mediterranean route presented similarities when it came to age, literacy, educational level, and life stories. The consequences of the journey and the way of perceiving themselves following the violence – not only sexual but also linked to emotional losses –undergone represented an obstacle against overcoming it with a view to disrupting the processes of resistance even when they seemed residual. The submissive and vilified body of many refugees/asylum seekers exerted powers of suggestion leading the way to more austere and anthropological fascination present in Mediterranean cultures related to male power within gender difference. For other interviewees – a few – the violence suffered at the hands of a proximate partner during particular phases of their lives was a condition of need fortunately not repeated.

The abridged excerpts provided above account for one-tenth of the interviews which were frequently cadenced by pauses and numerous silences transferring to terrible images and episodes of abuse, of physical and sexual violence difficult to bring to light. Some of them, like Ghana, burst into floods of tears. Others, on the other hand, told about their tragic little ruses. Among the asylum seekers interviewed the most common was that of pretending to be married to a particular man, whom they did not really know, so as to avoid having sex with strangers.

By comparing the stories of the interviewees, "the differences that make a difference" become evident (Crenshaw, 1991) when it comes to violent practices, and affect the construction of meanings. During the conduction of the interviews, in an all-female dynamic between interviewees and interviewers, the vulnerability of the interviewees became evident due precisely to the silences, the long pauses that punctuated stories that were vivid though barely sketched.

From the categories – abuse, deception, and proximity violence – that Ghana, Foluke, and Aziza represent, some accessory nodes were identified and developed with regard to particular cases of gender segregation and proximity violence which emerged during interviews with other migrant women hosted by the Palermitan SPRARS. One recurring attitude observed was general and uncritical acceptance of male domain by their female partners. Sometimes the researcher had to witness a veritable representation of "how to please your partner". All the interviewees – the married women in the presence of their husbands – described their dynamics as a couple in similar terms, all closely linked to rituals and roles preformed and internalized. Their behaviour patterns legitimized by tradition, normalization, and customs, were, for this reason, non-negotiable, making it difficult, for the operators at the host shelters to identify them. And it is precisely the difficulty that operators came across when seeking to intervene favourably regarding the hosting process which makes exposure to forms of violence "trivial". Furthermore, it normalized the configuration of the scenario of violence, of the situational dynamics inherent in family patterns in the daily practice of couples hosted in SPRAR centres or living in the *Ballarò* district where the survey was conducted.

> *I am the one who gets up first and, even here, I take care of everything my husband needs. I wash the clothes, often prepare food (the guests have a kitchen at their disposal) because the food distributed to us during meals is not always to his liking, then I go to pray with the other women with his permission.* (Gnima, 24 years old, Cameroonian)

> *The pocket money? No. My husband keeps it to buy phone cards or anything else like drink and sweet things. If I want something, I ask him and he usually says yes.*
>
> *If he gets angry with me it's my fault. It is I who cannot do everything and make him angry. Unfortunately, I often get sick and it would be much better if I could do what I should as a wife even if I'm sick ... but I can't.* (Satou, 28 years old, Congolese)

> *No, he doesn't want me to dress like the women here, he doesn't like it and he would be angry if I did. Nor do I want to. I prefer to see him quiet. We women are wives to make our husbands feel good ... otherwise what would my job be? That of quarrelling all the time? Of being beaten?* (Mouskaba, 26 years old, Zimbabwe)

For the majority of the interviewees, only repeated physical violence is considered abusive, while all other forms of abuse, from economic to symbolic, to sexual exploitation, are often perceived as justifiable behaviour by a man, to whom the authority to impose order within the relationship and make instrumental use of the woman to keep the intimate relationship stable, is granted.

> *If he hits me, I cry, but then I get over it. After all, some explosion in a family is normal. Even my father got angry and beat my mother ... but it happened every now and then. My father was a quiet man and my husband is also quiet.* (Saneba, 23, Sudanese)

> *No, the woman in Tanzania does not decide to have a child. Children are made at the behest of the men.* (Couma, 33 years old, Tanzanian)

In a set of excerpts from the interviews, the mechanisms of domination through symbolic violence (Bourdieu, 1998), its incorporation into the "habitus" of men and women, through "adaptive preferences" (Nussbaum, 2011), are evident. The realization of female subordination, reproduced by couples of the Islamic faith in daily life, is accompanied by a more general naturalization of gender segregation and, sometimes, of degradation of the body. The effects of sexist segregation which are also evident in terms of total lack of personal freedom, regularly undergone by the interviewees in their married lives, may be considered instrumental and homogeneous to all patriarchal models based on male domination. From what the witnesses narrated, the husband exercises the right to use the female body for sexual and procreative purposes. Violation of the partner's body is a male prerogative endorsed by tradition. But the more subtle effects of the culture of patriarchy are highlighted through female vulnerability which activates personal resistance devices within the context of proximity violence.

The non-directional interviews conducted with the sub-Saharan women hosted at the refugee reception centres initially risked reinforcing the vulnerability of the interviews by laying them bare, as it were. Despite the non-directional interviews required no precise answers or any stimulation by the interviewer, the stories were came to light with considerable difficulty. The narration became self-narration which, through a process of self-reflection, brought a negative kind of awareness to the surface. Each interviewee discovered "having been unable", "not having understood in time", having transformed the abuse endured into deception, into veritable delusion, mystification which, during the interviews, were progressively debunked and revealed in all their painful veracity. However, the help of the cultural intermediaries presents within the reception centres, and that of the members of the on-the-road help units who had longer contact than the authors with the Nigerian outdoor prostitutes, helped lower existing defensive barriers and foster true emotional interaction (Dahlberg, Dahlberg, & Nyström, 2008) from an insider–outsider perspective (Bonner & Tolhurst, 2002). If the co-presence of interviewer and interviewee highlighted the subjective vulnerability of the women interviewed (Fineman, 2008), this kind of vulnerability cannot be considered a characteristic intrinsic to either accounts, but as a trait characteristic of gender segregation tout court.

The risk taken, during the conduction of the non-directive interviews with the guests of the reception centres and migrants who live in the *Ballarò* district of Palermo, was that it might increase their vulnerability, by emphasizing elements that identified the lives of the interviewees. This risk could not be avoided even if we limited ourselves to taking note of the fragments of the stories, those episodes which, experienced first-hand, emerged during the interviewees' spontaneous flow of communication. Precisely the small number of prompt questions – 4 or 5 in all – by the interviewer, meant that the interviews managed to allow the interviewee to assess their own limit of tolerance with respect to their vulnerability/resistance. "It would seem that without being able to think about vulnerability, we cannot think about resistance, and that by thinking about resistance, we are already under way, dismantling the resistance to vulnerability in order precisely to resist" (Butler et al., 2016: 27).

2.5 Conclusions

To separate the issue of the proximity violence undergone by the sub-Saharan women, interviewed from the cultural representations used to explain it or from the processes of resilience and resistance that underscore it, would mean disjointing it from possible interpretations which "naturalize" it and lead to a kind of "racialization" of migrant women (Crenshaw, 1991; Razack, 2011).

From the interviews it emerges that for most of the interviewees only physical violence is considered truly violent, while all the other forms of ill-treatment, from economic to symbolic abuse, to sexual exploitation, are frequently perceived as justifiable behaviour on the part of males who are invested with the authority to establish order within the relationship and make instrumental use of women for the very purpose of maintaining their intimate relationship. The "bitter" contribution made by this research is that the man–woman dyad is delineated by what separates the other "authorized to", as husband, brother, father ... subject close to the victim, compared to the "unauthorized" stranger. A cultural substratum based on the concept of honour legitimizes the shame of proximity violence through the dyad of a subject, proximate person, and unauthorized foreigner (Bartholini, 2015) authorized to violate the body and, with it, the identity and personal integrity of a woman.

Therefore, one of the main problems surrounding gender-based violence and one which makes finding ways of impeding it difficult is that for most of the women interviewed, proximity violence is permissible, tolerated, and justified thanks to traditional views of the couple or because of emotional dependency. From this point of view, patriarchy (Edwards, 1987; Garcia-Moreno et al., 2006) is not simply an interpretative category of violence referring to the economic, cultural, or religious peculiarities of its actors, but finds its epistemic characterization in the kind of violence that victims undergo at the hands of close henchmen, as in the cases of Ghana's abuse-ridden journey, the exploitation of Foluke and Aziza's forced marriage. This is substantiated, at present, by means of the cross-grafting and strengthening of cultures of different origins due to the waves of migration, and expressed through the normalization of violence at the symbolic level. From the interviews conducted, it may be inferred that women perceive violence as a problem only when it degenerates and/or broadens the circle of its perpetrators beyond a proximity relationship which establishes the victim's submission to a sole subject.

The intersectional approach also highlighted how gender is a necessary but insufficient category by which to interpret dynamics and trajectories that are also influenced by the differences that each one of the women interviewed and every woman in general incorporates (Crenshaw, 1991; Nixon & Humphreys, 2010).

The prostitution of some of them also proves instrumentally useful to a certain kind of organized male crime market (Abbatecola, 2011; Kelly, 2005), but the abuses repeatedly suffered by other interviewees regarding even the context of married life may be considered equally instrumental and functional to patriarchal models based on abuse and male domination (Farmer, 2003). For other interviewees – only a few – the violence suffered at the hands of partners close to them during particular stages of their lives was a condition dictated by exigency and, fortunately, not reiterated in Italy.

It is necessary to keep in mind that the interviewees' pathway to self-awareness of their vulnerability was studded with pauses and numerous instances of sudden silence as they narrated their stories. During these pauses and silences, they recalled terrible images of abuse, of physical and sexual violence and found it difficult to reveal, even speak of them. Some of them like Ghana burst into uninterruptable floods of tears. For the sub-Saharan interviewees the most common ruse was to pretend being married to a certain man, whom they did not actually know, to avoid having sexual relations with strange men.

By comparing the interviewees' stories, "differences that make a difference" (Crenshaw, 1991) became evident in violent practices themselves and affected the construction of meanings and above all conditions capable of preventing them from overcoming proximity violence. The Latin word proximus is, grammatically speaking, an absolute superlative indicating the person closest to someone in a given space, at a given time (Bartholini, 2013). For the sub-Saharan women alike, it meant the link with a person close to them (usually a partner, but also the men on the boats, or the pimps with whom a useful link had been established) determining acceptance of the violence undergone within a particular context.

Although it is in no way easy to speak of sexual violence perpetrated by a stranger (Siegel & De Roos, 2016) the "bitter" contribution made by this survey is that the "friend–enemy" transforms the old dyad which opposed the proximus, who was "entitled to" because of being a husband, father, or brother, to him who was "not entitled to" because of being extraneous, So the friend–enemy dyad becomes the authorized-proximus versus the unauthorized-stranger (Bartholini, 2013) violating or not a woman's body and with it her personal identity and integrity. The "sweet" contribution is found in this very same vulnerability, which presupposes a certain degree of wife-victim, abused-fiancée, and lover-of-one-man-only – prostitute found in the testimonies of the sub-Saharan women. This vulnerability, initially discriminating in itself, as the interviews proceeded in an all-female gender-dynamic involving the interviewees and the interviewers, actually favoured a potential kind of caring empathy that identified the vulnerability of the victim for the sole purpose of mitigating it (Butler, 2004) and avoiding any kind of possible resistance.

In proximity violence it is symbolic and material oppression, culturally stratified and relationally embodied by the victim, which renders the victim acquiescent. This is due to the vulnerability of the victim, in one respect, but also because of that sentimental and/or fiduciary dependence, which turns vulnerability into resistance, adaptation to the situation and to the victim's own condition. It assumes the function of a cement within the dynamics that substantiate it. Within relationships involving it stabilizes the relationship.

Proximity violence unites a number of actions ranging from beatings to rape, to the physical elimination of the victim, from submission to slavery at both physical and symbolic levels, over a time span which allows the continuation of the violent act itself and its repetition to the bitter end. It reveals itself in relational contexts with a beginning and an end, which, in the worst case coincides with the destruction of the victim, negotiated, concerted as well as undergone by the weaker party, resistant to acknowledgement of the violence of which she was a victim, considering it "normal" or, at least, "not objectionable".

Resistance denotes conscious exposure to the victim's domination by the persecutor, and the attempt to resist it by facing up to the most deleterious effects, without however relieving oneself from that same dependence on the persecutor which favours violence as a normalized practice. From this angle, the resistance of a vulnerable subject does not permit her to overcome exposure to the power of the other, but underpins her permanence within the condition in which it is found (Butler, 2004; Butler et al., 2016). The reiteration of violence suffered is itself a consequence of the victim's resistance favouring the dynamics that make her the perpetrator's victim. Male domination, and the way in which it is not only imposed but leads to resistance on the part of the victim, means avoiding a condition/situation that she fails to acknowledge in all its gravity, precisely by virtue of the oppressive relationship that binds her to her abuser. It is intuitive to understand why resistance is tantamount to personal renunciation: the exposure of each of the interviewees to a triple form of subordination, imposed by their communities of origin, internalized during the migratory process, and, finally, reproduced in the countries where they require protection, does not seem to yield to any variant.

References

Abbatecola, E. (2011). *L'altra donna. Immigrazione e prostituzione in contesti metropolitani*. Milan, Italy: FrancoAngeli.

Bartholini, I. (2013). *Violenza di prossimità. La vittima, il carnefice, lo spettatore e il "grande occhio"*. Milan, Italy: FrancoAngeli.

Bartholini, I. (Ed.). (2015). *Violenza di genere e percorsi mediterranei. Voci, saperi, uscite*. Milan, Italy: Guerini e Associati.

Bartholini, I. (2016). Emancipazione pubblica privata. Tratteggi di una gender violence tardo moderna nell'incrociarsi di paradigmi atlantici e mediterranei. *Autonomie locali e servizio sociale, 2*(3), 56–81.

Bartholini, I. (2020). *The PROVIDE training course. Contents, methodology, evaluation*. Milan, Italy: FrancoAngeli.

Bernstein, E. (2007). Sex work for the middle classes. *Sexualities, X*(4), 472–488.

Bimbi, I. (2015). Onore-e-vergogna. Il ritorno di un paradigma mediterraneo nel dibattito europeo. In I. Bartholini (Ed.), *Violenza di genere e percorsi mediterranei. Voci, saperi, uscite* (pp. 27–44). Milan, Italy: Guerini e Associati.

Blumer, H. (1969). *Symbolic interactionism, perspective and method*. Englewood Cliffs, NJ: Prentice-Hall.

Bograd, F. (1999). Strengthening domestic violence theories: Intersections of race, class, sexual orientation, and gender. *Journal of Marital and Family Therapy, 25*, 275–289.

Bonner, A., & Tolhurst, G. (2002). Insider-outsider perspectives of participant observation. *Nurse Researcher, 2*, 9–19.

Bourdieu, P. (1998). *La nomination masculine*. Paris: Edition di Seul.

Bracke, S. (2016). Bouncing back: Vulnerability and resistance in times of resilience. In J. Butler, Z. Gambetti, & L. Sabsay (Eds.), *Vulnerability and resistance* (pp. 52–75). Durham, NC: Duke University Press.

Butler, J. (2004). *Undoing gender*. Abington, UK: Routledge.
Butler, J. (2016). Rethinking vulnerability and resistance. In J. Butler, Z. Gambetti, L. Sabsay (Eds.), *Vulnerability in resistance*. Durham: Duke University Press.
Butler, J., Gambetti, Z., & Sabsay, L. (2016). *Vulnerability in resistance*. Durham, NC: Duke University Press.
Coin, F. (2004). *Gli immigrati, il lavoro, la casa*. Milan, Italy: FrancoAngeli.
Collins, R. (2008). *Violence. A micro-sociological theory*. Princeton, NJ: Princeton University Press.
Connell, R. W. (2002). *Gender trouble*. Cambridge, UK: Polity Press.
Corbetta, P. (2015). *Metodologia e tecniche della ricerca sociale*. Bologna, Italy: il Mulino.
Corradi, C. (2009). *Sociologia della violenza. Modernità, identità, potere*. Rome, Italy: Meltemi.
Corradi, C., & Stöckl, H. (2016). The lessons of history. The role of the nation states and the EU in fighting violence against women in 10 European countries. *Current Sociology, 64*(4), 671–688.
Crenshaw, K. (1991). Mapping: Intersectionality, identity politics and violence against women of colour. *Standford Law Review, 43*, 124–129.
Crisp, J., Morris, T., & Refstie, H. (2012). Displacement in urban areas: New challenges, new partnerships. *Disasters, 36*(1), 23–42.
Dahlberg, K., Dahlberg, H., & Nyström, M. (2008). *Reflective lifeworld research*. Lund: Studentlitteratur.
De Wal, F. (1992). Intentional deception in primates. *Evolutionary Anthropology, 1*(3), 86–92.
Edwards, A. (1987). Male violence in feminist theory: An analysis of the changing conceptions of sex/gender violence and male dominance. In J. Hanmer & M. Maynard (Eds.), *Women, violence and social control. Explorations in sociology*. London: Macmillan.
Farmer, P. (2003). *Pathologies of power: Health, human rights, and the new war on the poor*. Berkeley, CA: University of California Press.
Ferrarotti, F. (1989). *La sociologia alla riscoperta della qualità*. Rome, Italy/Bari, Italy: Laterza.
Filosof, F. (2000). Violenza economica come contesto alla violenza domestica. In P. Romito (Ed.), *Violenze alle donne e risposte delle istituzioni* (pp. 39–48). Milan, Italy: FrancoAngeli.
Fineman, M. (2008). The vulnerable subject: Anchoring equality in the human condition. *Yale Journal of Law & Feminism, 20*(1/2), 1–23.
Garcia-Moreno, C., Jansen, H., Ellsberg, M., Heise, L., Watts, C. (2006), *Prevalence of intimate partner violence: findings from the WHO multi-country study on women's health and domestic violence*, Lancet, retrieved from https://www.ncbi.nlm.nih.gov/pubmed/17027732.
Gillioz, L., De Puy, J., & Ducret, V. (2000). La violenza domestica in Svizzera: nuovi dati su un fenomeno antico. In P. Romito (Ed.), *Violenze alle donne e risposte delle istituzioni* (pp. 83–96). Milan, Italy: FrancoAngeli.
Giordano, C. (1994). Der Ehrkomplex im Mittelmeerraum: sozialanthropologische Konstruktion oder Grundstruktur mediterraner Lebensform? In L. Vogt & A. Zingerle (Eds.), *Ehre. Archaische Momente in der Moderne* (pp. 172–192). Frankfurt a.M., Germany: Suhrkamp Verlag.
Gorman, G., Clayton, P., Shep, S., & Clayton, A. (2005). *Qualitative research for the information professional*. London: Facet Publishing.
Hajdukowski-Ahmed, M., Khanlou, N., & Moussa, H. (2009). *Not born a refugee woman: Contesting identities, rethinking practices*. New York/Oxford, UK: Berghahn.
Heller, A. (1985). *The power of shame: A rationalist perspective*. London: Routledge and Kegan Paul.
Herzfeld, M. (1980). Honour and shame: Problems in the comparative analysis of moral systems. *Man, XV*, 339–351.
Illouz, E. (2008). *Saving the modern soul: Therapy, emotions, and the culture of self-help*. Berkeley, CA: The University of California Press.
Jaji, R. (2009). Masculinity on unstable ground: Young refugee Men in Nairobi, Kenya. *Journal of Refugee Studies, 22*(2), 177–194.
Johnson, M. P. (2006). Conflict and control gender symmetry and asymmetry in domestic violence. *Violence Against Women, 12*(11), 1003–1018.

Kapur, R. (2002). The tragedy of victimization rhetoric: Resurrecting the native subject in international/post-colonial feminist legal politics. *Harvard Human Rights Law Journal, 15*, 1–32.

Kelly, L. (2005). 'You can find anything you want': A critical reflection on research on trafficking in persons within and into Europe. In F. Laczko & E. Gozdziak (Eds.), *Data and research on human trafficking: A global survey* (pp. 235–266). Geneva, Switzerland. Retrieved from: https://publications.iom.int/system/files/pdf/global_survey.pdf

Kirby, P. (2006). *Vulnerability and violence: The impact of globalization*. London: Pluto Press.

Krause-Vilmar, J. (2011). *Preventing gender-based violence: Building livelihoods. Guidance and tools for improved programming, Women's Refugee Commission*. Retrieved from: https://reliefweb.int/report/world/toolkit-optimizing-cash-based-interventions-protection-gender-based-violence

Macioti, M. I., & Pugliese, E. (2010). *L'esperienza migratoria: immigrati e rifugiati in Italia*. Rome, Italy/Bari, Italy: Laterza.

Mason, G. (2002). *The spectacle of violence*. London: Routledge.

Menjìavar, A., & Salcido, J. (2002). Immigrant women and domestic violence: Common experience in different countries. *Gender and Society, 16*(6), 898–920.

Nixon, J., & Humphreys, C. (2010). Marshalling the evidence: Using intersectionality in the domestic violence frame. *Social Politics, 17*, 137–158.

Nussbaum, M. (2000). *Women and human development: The capabilities approach*. Cambridge: University Press.

Nussbaum, M. (2011). *Creating capabilities: The human development approach*. Cambridge, MA: The Belknap Press of Harvard University Press.

Peano, I. (2013). Opaque loves: Governance and escape in the intimate sphere of Nigerian sex workers. *Etnografia e Ricerca Qualitativa, 3*, 359–384.

Peristiany, J. G. (Ed.). (1965). *Honor and shame: The values of Mediterranean society*. London: Weidenfeld & Nicolson.

Pinelli, B. (2011). Attraversando il Mediterraneo. Il "Sistema campo" in Italia: violenza e soggettività nelle esperienze delle donne. *Lares, 77*(1), 159–179.

Povinelli, E. (2002). Notes on gridlock: Genealogy, intimacy, sexuality. *Public Culture, 14*(1), 215–238.

Råheim, M., Magnussen, L., Sekse, R., Lunde, A., Jacobsen, T., & Blystad, A. (2016). Researcher–researched relationship in qualitative research: Shifts in positions and researcher vulnerability. *International Journal Qualitative Studies Health Well-being, 11*. Retrieved from https://www.ncbi.nlm.nih.gov/pmc/articles/PMC4910304/

Razack, S. (2011). *La chasse aux musulmans. Evincer les musulmans de l'espace politique*. Montréal, QC: Lux Éditeur.

Reale, E. (2000). Vita quotidiana delle donne: rischi di violenza e di disagio psichico. In P. Romito (Ed.), *Violenze alle donne e risposte delle istituzioni* (pp. 49–64). Milan, Italy: FrancoAngeli.

Romito, P. (2000). *La violenza di genere su donne e minori*. Milan, Italy: FrancoAngeli.

Schütz, A. (1967 [1932]). *The phenomenology of the social world*. Evanston, IL: Northwestern University Press.

Siegel, D., & De Roos, W. (2016). *Ethical concerns. Research on human trafficking*. New York: Springer.

Walby, S. (1990). *Theorizing patriarchy*. Cambridge, UK: Basic Blackwell.

Chapter 3
Human Trafficking: The Viscous Link Between Vulnerability and Proximity Violence

3.1 The Opaque Contours of Consent in Human Trafficking

Human trafficking is a phenomenon found worldwide and ranks among the highest on scales relating to international crime because of its diffusion and number of cases. It regards forced induction to various forms of exploitation, among which a prominent position is occupied by the exploitation of women for prostitution.

Italy is one of the European countries most affected by this phenomenon (OIM, 2017). A recent report by *Save the Children* (2019) reports that the phenomenon of trafficking for purposes of prostitution, which, in the past, regarded mainly women from non-European countries, today concerns women of Romanian nationality, mostly, as well as Albanians and Bulgarians, minors for the most part. According to the data of the European Commission, "between 2015 and 2016 [...], Italy counted 147 victims of Romanian origin, representing as much as 10% of the 1,511 victims of Romanian origin identified in the EU" (*Save the Children*, 2019: 26).

Although the common imagination tends not to differentiate between the foreign women involved in prostitution, the number of Romanian women who are victims of trafficking (51.6%) is clearly greater than that of Nigerian women (19%), while numbers are relatively low when it comes to married women (13.6%) or women with children (22.3%) (Ministero della Giustizia, 2015).

Every year in Italy, an average of 209 suits concerning human trafficking are registered with the offices of investigating magistrates, while an average of 33 appeals are registered annually with the Court of Assizes. The crime, in the cases registered, regards the sexual exploitation of women and minors and their concomitant induction into slavery. Human trafficking (punishable by art. 601 of the Italian Penal Code) represents 23% of a series of cases which goes hand in hand with reduction to slavery for a percentage of 73% (art. 600 of the Italian Penal Code), with alienation and the purchase of slaves (art. 602 of the Italian Penal Code) for a percentage of 4%. The law covers a long sequence of malicious acts including

I. Bartholini, *The Trap of Proximity Violence*,
https://doi.org/10.1007/978-3-030-52451-7_3

"recruitment, transportation [...] kidnapping, fraud, deception, abuse of power (...) for the purpose of exploitation" (art. 601 of the Italian Penal Code). The numbers of victims, referable to crimes registered in Italy, are, however, and with all probability, only a small part of a far vaster and more submerged phenomenon.

A similarly disturbing series of crime against the human person induces us to investigate, first of all, the mechanisms upstream of the exploitation and, in extreme cases, of the enslavement of another human being, which cannot have been determined exclusively for economic reasons. The *United Nations Protocol on the prevention, suppression, and persecution of human trafficking, in particular, of women and children* – commonly referred to as the "Palermo Protocol" – adopted by the United Nations Organization (UN) in Palermo in 2000, and which became effective in December 2003, made its international legislative adoption on the issue of trafficking in human beings possible.

It is defined as follows:

1. The "act" (recruitment, transport, transfer, hosting, or reception of people).
2. The "means" (the use or threat of the use of force or other forms of coercion, kidnapping, fraud, deception, abuse of position).
3. The "purpose" (the exploitation of prostitution by others or other forms of sexual exploitation, forced labour or services, slavery or similar practices, enslavement or organ harvesting).

However, the concept of "vulnerability" within the same Protocol as well as the adoption of concepts such as "consent" and "exploitation" may be simultaneously inclusive and exclusive, restrictive, and extensive, thus posing limits to interpretations of the definition of "victim of trafficking" in relation to "act, means, purpose" (Gallagher, 2010, 2012, 2015). In particular, the situational and contextual dimensions of personal vulnerability do not seem to have been attributed sufficient weight, to date, when defining the strategies permitting the subjugation of victims to their traffickers and lack of defence against them. The vulnerability of victims, even when exposed to a *vulnus* acknowledged at the legal level, does not *fully* explain the mechanisms which permit the permanent perpetration of their exploitation, especially when new situations and variables capable of providing for their release arise. The "means", as strategies implemented by the trafficker, play a fundamental role when it comes to the strongest keeping the weakest in a condition of dependence and exposure to violence, precisely by virtue of the context in which both parties find themselves and the interpersonal situation experienced.

Although the aforementioned directive describes vulnerability as a condition in which a person "has no other effective and acceptable choice than to give in to the abuse of which he is a victim" (art. 2), this condition is understandable only considering the context in which it is experienced and the situation that determines the "voluntary participation" in, as well as conditioning of victims to their own sexual exploitation. This means does not seem to find justification only in Weberian-type *Zweckrationalität*, which considers survival itself as the end that justifies the victims' submission, and consequent reification of their bodies by the perpetrator/trafficker.

Exploitation implies – and this is what will be discussed here – reasons of a different nature, in addition to purely economic and instrumental ones linked to the victim's own vulnerability.

Although a large number of stories indicate initial deception as the founding moment of their induction into slavery, the subsequent difficulty the victims encounter in acknowledging having been "forced and harassed" by one or more traffickers cannot be attributed exclusively to fear of an alien subject, but suggests that more complex and opaque degrees of emotional reluctance are at work within the strategies and practices used to exploit people. It is a matter – as we shall try to argue in the following pages – of relational aspects accompanied by an indirect, direct, symbolic and concrete violence, which could never have been produced by an exploiter/trafficker considered "alien" by the victims and to their emotional perception. And it is precisely in the stranger–neighbour dyad that the very possibility of procrastinating the sexual exploitation of the victims of trafficking by the trafficker in certain contexts and certain situations contributes to the identification of the "act", the "purpose", and above all the "means of abuse of power".

3.2 Vulnerability and Proximity Violence

3.2.1 Vulnerability

In recent years, vulnerability has been considered the "litmus test" by which to recognize the human rights of victims and, more specifically, of migrant victims (Fineman 2008, 2009). And this by the social sciences, which have contributed to identifying vulnerable subjects, and in by the law, which has qualified the subjects of legislation by confirming and expanding the obligations of the State in terms of social rights.

Vulnerability is a primarily contextual condition, strongly determined by institutions (Fineman 2010, 2016) that do not provide the resources which should permit the most fragile subjects to defend themselves. Secondly, vulnerability is situational, that is, it is determined by interpersonal relationships which reinforce the condition of vulnerability.

According to Penedo and Wrabetz (2015) there are three types of vulnerability:

1. Pre-existing, where vulnerability depends, above all, on the victim's background, including the physical and psychological condition of the individual, age, gender, pregnancy, culture, language, beliefs, and family condition.
2. Contextual, where a condition of vulnerability may be created or maintained, as in the case of one's administrative status within a territory, this kind of vulnerability may be generated or reiterated due to social, cultural, or linguistic marginalization.
3. Circumstantial, that is, created or maintained due to contingent events such as unemployment or economic indigence determined by supervening factors like illness.

This tripartition has been summed up well in the definition provided in 2008 by the UNODC according to which vulnerability is "a condition resulting from how individuals negatively experience the complex interaction of social, cultural, economic, political and environmental factors that create the context for their communities" (2008: 8).

However, even if this concept is identified in the above-mentioned tripartition, it is not always capable of interpreting the specific needs of individuals or groups, within particular contexts. Above all, it fails to identify, beyond the provision of a useful prima facie indication of the body's exposure to the *vulnus*, procedural strategies, intimate rituals, and relational arrangements that conceal far more complex implications that permit the victim to accept that very *vulnus* in situations and contexts peculiar. Similar strategies, adjustments, and rituals favour the emergence and persistence of a certain kind of emotional reluctance on the part of victims to recognize their own vulnerability. Furthermore, if the concept of vulnerability has been usefully addressed by political thinking when it comes to the human rights of some categories of subjects, it has also favoured less reflection on the causes that might induce one to seek freedom from a condition of slavery and exploitation of one rather than of another human being. Vulnerability cannot be considered, actually only as an intrinsic characteristic of the person (Fineman, 2008, 2016), but to be seen, rather, as "a part of the construction of situations and identities" (Butler, 2015: 228) which is defined also and above all within relationships of proximity where violence is constantly present. It is, therefore, a matter of highlighting the complex network of causes that determine the subjugation of a person, since violence not only acts upon but through bodies, in a blend of complicity, consent, and need for recognition by the victim. As Butler writes, "The very fact of being bound up with others establishes the possibility of being subjugated and exploited [...]. But it also establishes the possibility of being relieved of suffering, of knowing justice and even love" (2009: 61).

Several testimonies – of which we shall provide an account in paragraph 4 – describe initial deception accompanied by the victim's difficulty in recognizing the deception itself.

This allows us to hypothesize the emergence of opaque forms of emotional reluctance. This reluctance lies between the victims' resilience and their capacity for resistance, intended as both compensatory strategies which, if, on the one hand, favour the physical subordination of the exploited persons to the will of the trafficker, on the other, permits self-justification of dependence and subordination on the part of the victims. It is therefore a "pathogenic vulnerability" (Mackenzie, Rogers, & Dodds, 2014), that is, one dependent on a situation of oppression, favoured by a broader context, from which it becomes impossible to escape due to the directly or indirectly imposed violence itself. The latter constitutes the cement of the relationship between the victim and the trafficker. *Resilience*, in a context of deprivation and an interpersonal situation of oppression, needs to be seen as the creation of compensatory mechanisms within the situation experienced, *resistance* as the victims' ability to create a self-narrative of the violence undergone, which, in its mellowed form, makes the experience acceptable.

Therefore, the persistence of the victim in a condition of subordination may be attributed to a behavioural strategy that brings leverage to bear on the vulnerability of the victim within a situation which denotes, in any case, a degree of proximity violence such as to activate mechanisms of resistance. In other words, the victims become resistant to recognition of the proximity violence to which they are subjected even before becoming the victims of sexual exploitation by strangers.

To dwell, therefore, on the phenomenon of trafficking proves useful when seeking to draw up the *sui generis* script embodied by the victims, and with it, the recurring pattern of "the social order functioning as an immense symbolic machine aimed at ratifying the male domination on which it is based" (Bourdieu, 1998: 15), within contexts where the game of existence – sink or swim – is radicalized through the female body. The woman's body is the "primary place where violence is concretized" (Corradi, 2011: 11): the body is violated, abused. The human form – as Corradi writes – possesses a "symbolic power which surpasses any other sign" (Corradi, 2005: 9).

3.2.2 *Proximity Violence*

Almost all the relationships that make up an individual's universe of the senses incorporate a certain degree of epistemic (Spivak, 1990) and symbolic (Bourdieu, 1998) violence. By this is meant the product of the internalizations of constrictive social representations which define the cognitive structures of groups and/or populations, as well as individuals. This leads to "adaptive preferences" (Nussbaum, 2011), often based on erroneous beliefs or false interpretations of the facts.

Starting from this general assumption, proximity violence, in its symbolic makeup, is a phenomenon functional to the perpetuation of a system based on "social constructs" (Berger & Luckmann, 1966), referring to basic power relations between men and women. This means that it is legitimized through the production of meaning that makes specific behavioural patterns and attitudes recognizable within situations or "provinces of meaning". Within this "mutual game of structures of relevance" (Schütz, 1956) an object or event becomes the theme or topic of our thinking within a context which justifies it and shares its meaning.

In the relationship between victims and traffickers, the latter are not "neutral subjects", but "the" person or "one of" the persons legitimated by patriarchal codes to segregate the victims by placing them within his or her sphere of influence. Like a husband or brother acting within patriarchal contexts of pre-modern societies where women have no decision-making and self-management power, the trafficker becomes the "master" of the victim. Beyond any construction of power endorsed by the cultural context, however, acceptance of violence on the part of the victim, rendered possible within a rapport of dependence, even one of an emotional nature, becomes resistance against liberation of the victim from a condition of vulnerability even in the presence of favourable circumstances (Bartholini, 2018). The management of one's own person, entrusted to another who exercises power over one due to the asymmetrical position they occupy with respect to the victim and because victims are unable to find the independence and ability within themselves (to act, to narrate their lives as products of their own choices and projects), represents the victim's "hard core of fragility" (Ricoeur, 2007).

Furthermore, the story of a possible better future – imagined and outlined by the trafficker on behalf of the victim – is used as a lever by the trafficker to force the victim to accept the present as a necessary part of a plan aimed at improving their condition. The exploitation of the female body, after its initial sale, is rendered possible thanks to emotional dependence acting as a cement between the victim and the exploiter/trafficker. It acts as a veritable "test" of an "intimate contract" renewed through resistance against rejection of the methods used by the perpetrator to hetero-manage the victim's body. Trafficking, in itself, is the result of the victims' dependence/resistance against severing the dynamics that place them at the mercy of their exploiter/trafficker. Male domination, and the way in which it is not only imposed but undergone, refers to a paradoxical kind of subjection, an effect of what Bourdieu (1998) called symbolic violence; an invisible violence exercised by the dominator over the dominated to normalize the effects of given world views, social roles, cognitive categories, mental constructs, radicalized in patriarchies and in a sort of emotional-trust dependency dyad accompanying gender relationships.

The term *proximus* – "closest" – is a Latin superlative absolute denoting "the person closest to another", and may refer to a type of relationship where the subjects are connected, within a space–time dimension, which permits physical contiguity and exploitation of the victim, as well as intimacy. The *proximus* is most often the other who, in a relationship of physical, of situational proximity, therefore, occupies a dominant position. It is usually people who perceive themselves as most vulnerable who refer to or mention the *proximus*, and not vice versa. These relationships are victim–perpetrator or perpetrator-based, one where the other is not necessarily linked through sexual intimacy. Intimacy is one facet of proximity though it does not coincide totally with it. Proximity indicates a degree of situational closeness, which is detectable, nonetheless, on the basis of the degree of dependence and unconscious trust created and turned into a priori "consensus" granted by the victim to the perpetrator.

This dominance is almost always based explicitly on gender difference, on an asymmetry of power made official by family ties and/or legitimized by means of fiduciary agreements or real pacts, even of an economic nature. This kind of abuse of power is based, however and above all, on psychological manipulation often prior to exploitation, and perpetrated in an oppressive context, above all in a situation which renders vulnerable subjects open to proximity violence. The category of situational proximity, which throws light on the intimate nature of a relationship, makes all kinds of "abuse" of a victim possible. This method of exploitation may be extended even outside of the relationship. In the case of victims of trafficking, the possibility of being subjected to violence directly by the exploiter, but, above all, by third parties – customers – depends on the victim's trust, to a kind of blank delegation accorded by the victim to the oppressor. Violence is a particularly substantial risk for the majority of migrants, precisely because of the mestizament of exogenous and endogenous factors in their lives; it does not regard asymmetry of power alone but the context in which it is structured and the situation which emerges as an intervening variable. In the case of female migrants, victims of trafficking, it is a matter of evaluating four indicators:

1. The material conditions that define the victims' the daily lives (contexts).
2. The subjective dimension which renders some of them more exposed to violence (passive vulnerability).
3. Sudden events intentionally created by the trafficker which aggravate the already precarious condition of victims, making them more exposed to abuse of power (active vulnerability).
4. Relationships of proximity (situations) created contingently and which assume violence as a modality proper to relationships between traffickers and their victims, permitting the abuse of power to act as a "means" itself.

Proximity violence takes place and is strengthened only in the presence of the aggregation of subjective variables which induce the victim to transform their vulnerability into surrender to their perpetrators of their very persons (Bartholini, 2018, 2019) who can then manipulate them. In similar situations, the exploiter is "that" *proximus* who is part of the emotional experience of victims who define their identities in relation to the other and, consequently, permit the identification of the other to be reflected in that particular situation which provides for the unleashing of an emotional surplus. No victim of trafficking would accept selling herself to a series of men, if this experience were not shared indirectly by the trafficker, unless he were aware of the abnormal circumstances being experienced by the victim, thus providing victim with the illusion that he is aware of the discomfort to which he is exposing her.

This means that the victim's acceptance of the direct and indirect proximal violence undergone cannot be attributed solely to the vulnerability which delivered her to the trafficker, but rather to the intrinsic mechanisms of proximity which shape emotional dependence accompanied by resilience and resistance, which render the victim docile and inclined to normalize violence even in the presence of a way out.

The abuse perpetrated as a result of a voluntary acceptance by victims is subject to the degree of proximity violence that has been metabolized and normalized between the abuser and the abused within the relationship. Normality/normalization can only be explained by identification of indicators capable of explaining its dynamics. Unlike gender-based violence, proximity violence is based on a precise pact made within a relationship; this pact clouds instrumental rationality and blurs the exploitation existing within this relationship of trust. Proximity violence is part of a self-sufficient, auto-immune rapport which excludes conflict.

1. Violence acts both as an instrument used to regulate relationships and as an autonomous social force capable of bestowing meaning on reality. As a structuring force of a relationship, it assigns the participants with tasks and roles within a commercial pact based on essential, emotional values which bind the contracting parties.

2. Since violence – in different forms and ways – becomes the very bond of the relationship, it assumes the characteristics of self-sufficiency. A type of violence, that is, which "suffices" to keep the relationship going.
3. This relationship based on violence excludes all and every form of resistance to violence, making the latter indispensable to maintaining the relationship which is auto-immune (Bartholini, 2013).

Were the logic of proximity violence separated from the use of "means" in specific contexts and situations, this would be tantamount to separate it from all possible interpretations capable of "naturalizing" it, thus producing a sort of "racialization" of migrants (Crenshaw, 1991; Razack, Smith, & Thobani, 2011).

3.3 The Framework Regulating the Concept of Vulnerability in Italy and Rumania

Both Romania and Italy, as Member States of the European Union, are obliged to incorporate into their national juridical norms Directive 2011/36/EU of the European Parliament and of the Council of 5 April 2011, "concerning the prevention and repression of trafficking of human beings and the protection of victims, and which replaces the Council Framework Decision 2002/629/JHA". Its Article n. 2 binds EU Member States to take "the necessary measures to punish the following malicious acts: the recruitment, transportation, transfer, accommodation or reception of people, including the passage or transfer of the authority over these people, with the threat of use or with the use of force or other forms of coercion, with the kidnapping, fraud, deception, abuse of power or vulnerable position or with the offer or acceptance of sums of money or benefits to obtain the consent of one person who has authority over another, for exploitation purposes" (Castelli, 2014).

In February 2014, the new penal code became effective in Rumania with the introduction of the crime of human trafficking (art. 210 of the Rumanian Penal Code) which referred to "the recruitment, transportation, transfer, accommodation or reception of people for the purpose of exploitation, through means of coercion, kidnapping, deception or abuse of power; or to take advantage of the inability to defend themselves or to express their will or particularly vulnerable status; through the offer or acceptance of sums of money or benefits to obtain the consent of a person who has authority over another".

In Italy, the crime of human trafficking is punishable according to art. 601 of the Penal Code which provides for a ruling of between eight to twenty years' imprisonment for whoever recruits, introduces into the territory of the State, or transfers outside it, exerts authority over a person, hosts one or more people in the conditions referred to in Article 600, that is, acts in the same way towards one or more persons, by means of deception, violence, threat, abuse of authority, or exploitation of a situation of physical, mental vulnerability or of necessity, by promising or bestowing money or other advantages on the person over whom they have authority, with a view to inducing or forcing them to work, perform sexual services, beg or, in any case, to carry illegal activities involving their exploitation or force them to undergo the removal of organs.

While the Italian Penal Code refers to the concept of victim vulnerability in relation precisely to the crime of human trafficking, the Romanian legal system, in art. 6 of law 292/2011, defines as vulnerable "individuals or families who are at risk of losing their ability to face daily due to illness, disability, poverty, addiction to alcohol or drugs or other situations that can lead to an economic or social vulnerability or people over 65".

The concept of vulnerability is, therefore, central to the evaluation of cases of human trafficking, and substantially refers to particular characteristics like age, gender, disability, race, or ethnicity which make certain individuals more inclined to become the victims of trafficking, especially if they belong to minorities who have no power to assert their rights. Membership of so-called *vulnerable groups* usually has its attractions for traffickers, who tend to choose their victims according to their degrees of vulnerability.

The *Explanatory Report of the Warsaw Convention* is the only official document which provides a more detailed interpretation of the concept, defining vulnerability as "any kind, whether physical, psychological, emotional, family-related, social or economic. The situation might, for example, involve the insecurity or illegality of the victim's administrative status, economic dependence, or fragile health. In short, the situation can be any state of hardship in which a human being is impelled to accept being exploited" (European Council, 2005). Although the definition provided by the European Council is redundant to some extent, it does manage to underline some concrete aspects, including emotional and family vulnerabilities (Pascoal, 2017). This particular reference of the Report introduces the idea of a kind of proximal vulnerability resulting from the convergence of contextual and situational conditions.

The notion of "proximal" vulnerability, illustrated in paragraph 2 by Ignazia Bartholini, include a whole series of situations where traffickers establish a relationship of trust, when not of a sentimental nature, with the victims, capable of conditioning their consent and blurring the boundaries between coercivity, opportunity, contextual necessity, and situational preference.

For the precise purpose of explaining this convergence, in the *Vulnerability Paper Issue* (Gallagher, 2012) published by the *United Nations Office on Drugs and Crime* – hereinafter indicated as UNODC – the Moldovan authorities highlighted the importance of the "means" permitting exploitation of vulnerable victims (the "act") for economic purposes (the "purpose"). By "means" was meant abuse of a position of vulnerability (APOV). It is through evaluation of the "means" that it is possible to establish degrees of coercion of victims. This assessment becomes fundamental in cases where it is not possible to detect "hard means" like the use of force and kidnapping.

APOV may also occur in cases where traffickers use "soft means" against vulnerable subjects, that is, strategies which are not immediately visible like deception and coercion (UNODC 2018).

The abuse against victims, as conceived by the Moldovan authorities, is made possible thanks to interactions of proximity, where situations and contexts favour the implementation of the "means of APOV". They bring leverage to bear on a situational, therefore, proximal condition of vulnerability, where violence is not necessarily acted upon, but is present within the indirect dynamics of the relationship. For this reason, perpetrators avail themselves of the knowledge they have of the victims in order to evaluate their weaknesses on which to exert leverage capable of facilitating their exploitation. Furthermore, "abuse of the vulnerable position" not only permit traffickers to exploit their victims, but also establishes the exploiters' hegemony, which tends to prolong the "deception" related to the effective and mutual emotional involvement between the victims and their exploiters/traffickers who are usually such only from the point of view of the victims. Consequently, by virtue of this "emotional deception", the subjects are unaware of being victimized, and this favours their sexual exploitation (Gallagher et al., 2017).

Therefore, as already highlighted by Bartholini, it is necessary to resort to the notion of situational and contextual vulnerability, to understand the real meaning of APOV and, therefore, the link between forms of passive vulnerability inherent in victims and active vulnerability, that is, forms intentionally created by traffickers (Pascoal, 2017), by means of mechanisms of trust established within the proximal relationship itself existing between the victims and the traffickers (Pascoal, 2017).

3.4 A Reading of Some Rulings of the Italian and Romanian Supreme Courts[1]

3.4.1 Some Methodological Considerations

The *Global Report on Trafficking in Persons* of the UNODC foregrounds the relevance of court rulings to analysis of "the patterns and flows of trafficking in persons" (UNODC 2018: 15), with a view to discouraging the perpetration of the phenomenon.

In order to describe the heterogeneity of the different interpretations of the concept of vulnerability that compete with other "soft means" like "deception" and "coercion" (Gallagher, 2010), we examined 22 rulings passed by the Italian Supreme and relating to art. 601 of the Italian Penal Code, drawing on the Pluris[2] and De Jure[3] legal platforms, and 35 regarding art. 210 of the Rumanian Penal Code, pronounced by the Romanian Supreme Court of Penal Law.[4] Of the initial 22 sentences,

[1] I thank Dr. Rafaela Pascoal who collaborated in identifying the Italian and Romanian sentences.

[2] http://pluris-cedam.utetgiuridica.it/main.html

[3] https://dejure.it/#/home

[4] https://www.scj.ro/, R O M Â N I A ÎNALTA CURTE DE CASAŢIE ŞI JUSTIŢIE Secţia Penală Decizia.

all passed during the same three-year period – 2015–2018 – those (7 in all) which involved Romanian women as victims of trafficking were selected, while 5 sentences passed by the Romanian Supreme Court were chosen to bestow greater relevance upon this paragraph.

A textual analysis was carried out using the NVivo 12 software (Non-numerical Unstructured Data Indexing, Searching and Theorizing Vivo), which acted as a fundamental working tool during the entire course of the textual analysis of the sentences. By using this software as a kind of hypertext to draw up a Document System comprising a number of conceptual nodes, it was possible to manage the coding, that is, the attribution of codes to segments of text referable to the contents of the rulings. The clarity of the goals we sought to achieve, availing ourselves of the material analysed, permitted us to expand the Node Browser, thus obtaining a vision more thorough than that provided by the coded text. In addition, the Non-numerical Unstructured Data Indexing, Searching and Theorizing Vivo favoured memorization of the steps followed during the analytical procedure and the choices made to facilitate interpretation of the research material.

The NVivo 12 software facilitated the following:

- identification and examination of the nodes
- identification of textual fragments within a node
- formulation of the queries, which make comparison between results over time fruitful

The nodes identified numbered 16, the textual fragments 218. Below are the frequencies of the text excerpts referring to the first 8 nodes, and which permitted us to describe the very core of the textual analysis carried out (Table 3.1).

On the whole, and as will emerge from the thorough examination provided in the next paragraph when the segments referring to the contents of the rulings are examined, greater attention is paid to the word "vulnerability" as "passive vulnerability" – also emerging with reference to issues regarding "age" and "economic condition" – of the victim as a precondition favouring exploitation. The Italian rulings appear to foreground the victims' linguistic difficulties, above all, "moral poverty" as an element preventing the victims from freeing themselves from their condition. The use of means as a key instrument of victim submission appears with

Table 3.1 The presence and numerical frequency of the nodes in the rulings analysed

Node	Rumanian rulings	Italian rulings
1st node: presence of the term "vulnerability"	14 times	5 times
2nd node: presence of the term "violence" (*loverboy method*)	9 times	2 times
3rd node: presence of the terms "means" and "APOV means"	14 times	17 times
4th node: linguistic and cultural difficulties	6 times	12 times
5th node: victim's age	16 times	8 times
6th node: economic difficulties	15 times	8 times
7th node: emotional addiction	6 times	14 times
8th node: moral poverty	3 times	11 times

similar frequency in the texts of the rulings of the Supreme Courts of both countries though with different degrees of sensitivity: the Romanian Court uses the term "loverboy method" frequently while the Italian rulings opt for the term "emotional addiction".

3.4.2 *An Analysis of Some Rulings Pronounced by Italian and Romanian Courts of Penal Law*[5]

A closer reading of the rulings themselves highlighted some differences in the assessment of the concept of vulnerability between the country of origin and the country of destination of the Romanian victims. This analysis of the rulings intended understanding how definitions of human trafficking were related by the courts to the concepts of "means", "purpose" and "act" within particular situations and contexts, at an intersection between endogenous and exogenous factors.

If when it came to "purpose" and "act" as dealt with in the rulings examined, no particular food for thought emerged, the examination of the "means" was, in our case, particularly charged, however, with weighty significance. Identifiable "means" were associated in the texts with specific strategies aimed at the trafficking and manipulation of victims by traffickers which revealed veritable practices of "abuse of a position of vulnerability", "deception", and "coercion".

The generalized use of the loverboy method emerged above all: a strategy aimed at the recruitment and sexual exploitation of the victim on the basis of a sentimental and fiduciary relationship between the trafficker and a vulnerable subject. This strategy appears to have received considerable acknowledgement in the Romanian rulings. This is the case of Ruling n° 131/RC/2016 pronounced by the Romanian Supreme Court, which clearly shows how the trafficker abused the victim's position of vulnerability to deceive and reprimand her constantly. She was only 16 years old, pregnant and in love with her exploiter. "[...] during the trial he also tried to use the same methods he availed himself of when he inducing the victim to prostitute herself, assuring her he would marry her and recognize the child if she gave him a hand".[6]

---

[5]This paragraph was written with the collaboration of Dr. Rafaela Pascoal of the University of Palermo whom I thank for having identified the sentences to which I refer in this chapter.

[6]"*Acesta, deşi aflat în stare de arest preventiv, a trimis părţii vătămate scrisori, prin care, profitând de starea vulnerabilă în care se afla, urmare a vârstei de doar 16 ani şi a stării de graviditate, folosindu-se de aceleaşi metode pe care le-a folosit şi pe parcursul desfăşurării activităţii infracţionale, respectiv declarându-i că o iubeşte, că se va căsători cu ea, că îi va recunoaşte copilul, i-a solicitat să revină asupra declaraţiilor date în cursul urmăririi penale şi să îl ajute în acest fel să scape de acuzaţii*" ["He, although in a state of preventive arrest, sent letters to the injured party, taking advantage of her vulnerable state, because she was only 16 and pregnant, using the same methods as those he already used during his criminal activity, that is, declaring his love for her, saying he would marry her, recognize the child and asking her to review the statements given during the criminal proceedings and help him to be freed from these accusations"], in https://www.scj.ro/1093/Detalii-jurisprudenta?customQuery%5B0%5D.Key=id&customQuery%5B0%5D.Value=130996, 10/06/2019.

The emotional dependence of the victim, created intentionally by the trafficker, was recognized as a "means" aimed at increasing the victim's subjection also in Ruling No. 134/A/2018 of the Romanian Supreme Court, which recites textually that "the use" of coercive psychological action, through the creation of emotional dependency for the purpose of exploitation "is known".[7]

Furthermore, in the same rulings passed by the Romanian Supreme Court, the expression *lipsa de experiență de viață* ("lack of life experience") associated with the age of the victim is reported several times as one of the most frequently considered factors. Highlighting the age of the victim is of fundamental importance when it comes to punishing the crime. Indeed, as established by the Palermo Protocol, that the minor age of a victim does not require the use of any further "means" to obtain the condemnation of the perpetrator, since minor age in itself places the victim in a position of inferiority with regard to the trafficker, and automatically excludes any possibility that the victim was consenting.

The judges of the Romanian victim's country of origin revealed that they were generally aware of "means" meant as "abuse of position of vulnerability" (APOV), especially in cases of victims from a context of material deprivation and cultural poverty associated with a lack of family care. In Ruling n° 162/RC/2016 of the Romanian Court, the judges stated verbatim that "the traffickers exploited the innocence of the victims and their vulnerabilities determined by the minor age and their relatively poor and disrupted family contexts. Initially, they were kind to the victims, to gain their trust and subdue them to the point where the minors themselves would have accepted prostituting themselves and being treated as objects".[8]

In Italy, too, the age of a victim is considered an important feature of passive vulnerability along with determinants relating to context. This is the case in Ruling n°. 5704 of 22/10/2018 of the Italian Supreme Court, which states that "child victims of trafficking were in conditions of vulnerability due to their age and lack of means of sustenance, reference and support" (Supreme Court of Penal Law – Sez. V, Ruling, n. 5703, dep. Il 05/02/2019).

---

[7] "*În cauză, acțiunea de racolare a victimelor, profitând de (...) și folosirea ulterior a actelor de constrângere psihică prin punerea victimelor într-o stare de dependență emoțională față de ei în scop de exploatare*" ["In this case, the action of restraining the victims, taking advantage of (...) and the subsequent use of acts of mental constraint by placing the victims in a state of emotional dependence on them for the purpose of exploitation"], in https://www.scj.ro/1093/Detalii-jurisprudenta?customQuery%5B0%5D.Key=id&customQuery%5B0%5D.Value=145672, 9/06/2019.

[8] "*au exploatat practic naivitatea și vulnerabilitatea acestora, datorată vârstei dar și problemelor familiale, comportându-se inițial frumos cu acestea, după* cum *au declarat chiar persoanele vătămate, promițându-le că le vor ajuta, câștigându-le practic încrederea, pentru ca apoi să le aducă în poziția de a le lua aproape toți banii câștigați în urma activităților de prostituție, tratându-le ca pe simple obiecte* ["they have practically exploited their naivety and vulnerability, due to their age but also to their family problems, initially behaving nicely to them, as the injured persons themselves have stated, promising to will help them, gaining their confidence, so that they may then be able to take almost all the money earned through prostitution treating them as mere objects"], in https://www.scj.ro/1093/Detalii-jurisprudenta?customQuery%5B0%5D.Key=id&customQuery%5B0%5D.Value=134631

If passive vulnerability appears primarily determined, in the texts of the rulings analysed, by the absence of a caring family and by a deprived socio-economic context, active vulnerability is found in the effects of emotional and physical submission deriving from the manipulative strategies implemented by the trafficker in an intimate context of emotional dependence and proximal violence. As a result, the victim ends up finding herself without an alternative except that of accepting the trafficker's offer of collaborating actively in the achievement of certain purposes that appear shareable. Economic deprivation and lack of parental care counterbalance cultural poverty and, sometimes, the failure of the victims to develop morally. Ruling n° 193/RC/2017 of the Romanian Supreme Court of Penal Law described a victim as "characterized by the lack of elementary values, leading to acceptance of acts of corruption typical of her position".[9] The economic and moral deprivation of victims was also highlighted by the Italian judges, who tended to add other specific socio-cultural factors of vulnerability like victims' lack of knowledge of the host country's language. This was the case of the Italian Supreme Court of Penal Law's Ruly n° 32322, where the judge acknowledged how the state of the victims' subjection was "fuelled by the condition of psychic inferiority in which they found themselves (in a land foreign to them, in conditions of poverty, without income and unable to express themselves in the Italian language)" (Ruling of the Supreme Court of Penal Law – Sez. III n° 32322, dep. of the 23/07/2015). In a context of situational vulnerability, the state of necessity of the victim was intended as "any situation of weakness or material or moral lack on the part of the passive person, which favours the conditioning of her personal will; this situation coincides essentially with her position of vulnerability" (Ruling of the Supreme Court of Penal Law – Section V n°. 8545 dep. on 27/02/2019).

In the court hearing of case no. 193/RC/2017, the General Directorate of Social Services and the Protection of Minors of the town of Iesi presented a psychological assessment of the victim, proving how the psychological damage highlighted in her case had been caused by a multiplicity of maltreatment and abuse of different kinds "stabilized" within a relationship of trust between the trafficker and his victim. In preliminary Ruling no. 331/RC/2017 of the Romanian Supreme Court, we read that the victim's mother stated that "the daughter had been diagnosed with a form of mental instability and emotional lability"[10] which aggravated the charges of trafficking against the defendant.

[9] "*profilul moral-educativ al victimei, marcat de lacune esențiale în privința unor valori cu caracter axiomatic-ca adevărul*"["the moral-educational profile of the victim, marked by essential gaps regarding axiomatic values – like the truth"], in https://www.scj.ro/1093/Detalii-jurisprudenta?customQuery%5B0%5D.Key=id&customQuery%5B0%5D.Value=145706

[10] R O M Â N I A ÎNALTA CURTE DE CASAȚIE ȘI JUSTIȚIE Secția Penală Ruling n.331/RC/2017, Ședința publică din 14 septembrie 2017 "*Prin declarația dată în fața inculpatului A. la data de 13 august 2007, martora B. a declarat că fiica a fost diagnosticată cu structură psihică instabilă, labilitate emoțională și că din verificările sale, aceasta „avea o relație cu un anume C., care locuiește în Brăila, și este plecată cu acesta în Spania*" ["According to the statement regarding defendant A. on August 13th, 2007, witness B. stated that her daughter had been diagnosed with unstable mental make-up emotional lability and that according to checks, she had a relationship with a certain C., living in Brăila, and now away with him in Spain"].

The exercise of proximity violence from the most explicit to the softest degrees of manipulation of the victim is counterbalanced by the situational and contextual vulnerability of the victims. This was noted, for example, in the Ruling of the Supreme Court, Penal section V, n° 34403 dep. of the 06/08/2015, where the investigating judge said that the exploitation "was based on the condition of absolute necessity of the very young girl, already a mother and without any means of support. M. was a 'friend of the family', and, therefore, well informed regarding the real conditions of weakness (psychological and economic) of I. and, therefore, of her state of vulnerability". Proximity violence, which also limits the victim's self-determination indirectly when it comes to the possibility of reporting her exploiter to the law. So much so, that Ruling n° 42751 of the Supreme Court of Penal Law sect. V dep of the 19/09/2017 highlighted the fact that "for the configurability of the crime of enslavement, total denial of personal freedom is not necessary, but a significant compromise of the capacity of self-determination of the offended person is sufficient to configure the relevant state of subjection for the purpose of integrating the incriminating norm". Furthermore, in the same Ruling it is highlighted that, despite the fact that "the Romanian young women could go out to go to the place of prostitution and return without a nagging 'escort', and that they were equipped with mobile phones, excludes asphyxiating control over customers' performance and entertainment times. This situation, as well as the obligation at ever heavier times and the immediate requisition of the sums in view of an unlikely future distribution, account for a more 'psychological' than 'physical' connotation of the awe of the girls". The exercise of proximity violence, from the most explicit to the softest degrees of manipulation of the victim, is counterbalanced by the situational and contextual vulnerability of the victims. This was noted, for example, in Ruling n° 34403 dep. on 06/08/2015 of Penal section V of the Supreme Court where the investigating magistrate held that exploitation had been "based on the condition of absolute necessity of the young girl, on the fact that she was already a mother and had no means of support. M. was a "friend of the family's", and, therefore, well-informed regarding I.'s real conditions of (psychological and economic) weakness".

Proximity violence also limits victims' self-determination indirectly when it comes to the possibility of reporting their exploiters. So much so, that Ruling n° 42751 of the Italian Supreme Court of Penal Law sect. V dep of the 19/09/2017 stated that "for the configurability of the crime of enslavement, total denial of personal freedom is not necessary, but a significant compromise of the offended person's capacity of self-determination is sufficient for the configuration of the relevant state of subjection with a view to integrating the incrimination". Furthermore, the Ruling emphasized the fact that the "young Romanian women could go out to their patches and return without a nagging 'escort', and that they were equipped with mobile phones which excluded asphyxiating control over customers' times of performance and enjoyment". This situation, as well as the obligation to provide increasingly longer times and the immediate requisition of the sums earned in view of some unlikely future distribution, account for a "psychological" rather than a "physical" connotation of the subjection of the girls.

3.5 Final Consideration

Despite the formulation of a definition of human trafficking at the international level, through the adoption of the Palermo Protocol, the application of "means" in rulings appears heterogeneous in its interpretation and adoption. Furthermore, the application of this definition tends to differ precisely in the rulings pronounced in countries both of origin and destination regarding victims of trafficking. However, it is exactly in the establishment of a balance between stable or stabilized factors (context and situation of proximal violence) and intervening variables ("act", "purpose" and, above all, "means"), that the phenomenon of trafficking becomes more readily identifiable.

Vulnerability is not inherent only in the corporeality of the human being (Fineman, 2008) and, although "we cannot understand it outside our corporality [...] it is located in human relationships" (Butler et al. 2016: 16). Bodily fragility, material needs, and dependence on the other are conditions proper to the human being which cannot be ignored when judging a crime.

As a result, analyses of the phenomenon of trafficking cannot take place without in-depth analyses of the use of "means" which, however, does not always receive adequate recognition in the rulings of the Supreme Courts. Furthermore, interpretations at the penal level sometimes diverge between the rulings of the recruiting and host countries, making associations between vulnerability and proximity violence viscous, thus, obscuring correct identification of the victims' submission and strategies of abuse.

In the cases analysed here, the Romanian judges attributed enormous importance to the victims' socio-cultural circumstances, both before and during recruitment, while balancing their active and passive vulnerabilities. The Italian judiciary tended, instead, to view vulnerability as the outcome of the contingent manipulation undergone by the victims in Italy. The vulnerability inherent in their initial condition and that produced subsequently through congeries of the phenomena of proximal violence should be considered, however, in the same way by the courts of both countries. In both instances, it appears to be a matter of a "situational" kind of vulnerability grafted onto circumstances of deprivation where the APOV is recognized as the "means" par excellence. It is a (passive) vulnerability which, in the countries of origin is the result of social exclusion, material poverty, and ignorance of the legal norms of the victims' countries of arrivals. It is an (active) type of vulnerability created within a situation of proximal violence, which induces victims to "rely on a stranger who has become close" (Bartholini, 2019: 26) who exercises the "means of abuse" directly and otherwise. A contextual vulnerability referable equally to the country of destination and produced by lack of contact with the local community, by linguistic difficulties, by the poverty of social relations (and here too we are in a situation of deprivation), but which would not have the same devastating power unless it were combined with the victims' emotional dependence on their traffickers (a situation emerging within a dynamic of proximity violence). The *vulnus* is hidden within the folds of the (false) consent given by victims to prostitute themselves, a kind of consensus determined by the proximal violence to which victims are subjected (Bartholini, 2013, 2018). This type of violence, being intimate and negotiable only within the relationship, determines a degree of manipulation ("means") which alters the emotional response of victims, turning distrust into trust, abuse into passion, exploitation of one's own body into a tool for the achievement of a presumed substantial improvement to one's life to be shared with the perpetrator. The inability of victims of trafficking to oppose abuse is not something produced by the victims' economic and cultural poverty alone, but, and above all, by emotional submission to and manipulation by the exploiter who creates voluntary forms of subordination and dependence (Bartholini, 2019). Therefore, active vulnerability may be read as a complex set of factors, calculated and provoked by the exploiter for utilitarian purposes, which lead to acceptance of abuse, in a regime of primary needs, justified by the situation, as well as by the contexts in which victims come to find themselves.

Precisely by virtue of the viscous links between violence of proximity and active and passive vulnerability, the concept of "means" of "abuse of a position of vulnerability" should be given even greater validity when bringing to the surface the situational factors which lead victims to subjection and which have been underestimated at the legal level for too long. This is especially true of cases where the traffickers use ambiguous strategies, where the victims' vulnerability and manipulation by the exploiter are not clearly evident (Gallagher et al., 2017). The detection of the crime of trafficking, unlike other types of crime concerning even a single criminal offence, is a complex and delicate procedure. It could be facilitated if the competent bodies brought leverage to bear on sets of factors like the victims' backgrounds, the active and passive vulnerabilities of which they are the bearers, the situation that has arisen between them and their traffickers, the proximity violence permeating the situation itself. These factors would make it possible to probe the temporal sequencing of the victimization of vulnerable subjects: "recruitment, transport [...] kidnapping, fraud, deception, abuse of power (...) for the purpose of exploitation" (Directive 2011/36/EU art.2) with a view to obtaining acknowledgement of the crime in both the countries of origin and of arrival.

In cases of exploitation, the power of the judiciary can correct, by recognizing the situational vulnerability and the "means" brought into play by the perpetrators, the way distortions, determined by the institutions which fail to acknowledge a crime, prevent victims from freeing themselves from trafficking.

References

Bartholini, I. (2013). *Violenza di prossimità. La vittima, il carnefice e il "grande occhio"*. Milan, Italy: FrancoAngeli.

Bartholini, I. (2018). The system hotspot: Politics of refusal against the economic migrants and absence of good practices for contrasting the gender and sexual violence suffered by migrants. In F. Pattaro Amaral, I. Bartholini, & R. Di Rosa (Eds.), *Migrations: A global welfare challenge: Policies, practices and contemporary vulnerabilities* (pp. 43–67). Barranquilla, Colombia: Ed. Corunamerica.

Bartholini, I. (2019). The phenomenology of proximity violence: Relational strategies and modalities used against vulnerable migrants. In I. Bartholini (Ed.), *Proximity violence in Migration times. A focus in some Regions of Italy, France and Spain* (pp. 31–50). Milan, Italy: Franco Angeli.

Berger, P., & Luckmann, T. (1966). *The social construction of reality*. London: Anchor.

Bourdieu, P. (1998). *La domination masculine*. Paris, France: Edition di Seul.

Butler, J. (2009). *Frames of war: When is life grievable?* London: Verso.

Butler, J. (2015). *Notes toward a performative theory of assembly*. Cambridge, MA: Harvard University Press.

Butler, J., Gambetti, Z., & Sabsay, L. (2016). *Vulnerability in resistance*. Durham, NC: Duke University Press.

Castelli, V. (2014). *Punto e a capo sulla tratta. Uno studio sulle forme di sfruttamento di esseri umani in Italia e sul sistema di interventi a tutela delle vittime*. Milan, Italy: Franco Angeli.

Corradi, C. (2005). *Il nemico Intimo. Una lettura sociologica dei casi di Novi Ligure e Cogne*. Rome, Italy: Meltemi.

Corradi, C. (2011). L'amore come istituzione totale. Un modello interpretativo della violenza contro le donne. *Spazio Filosofico, 3*, 1–12.

Crenshaw, K. (1991). Mapping the margins: Intersectionality, identity politics, and violence against women of color. *Stanford Law Review, 43*(6), 1241–1299.

European Council. (2005). *Explanatory report to the Council of Europe convention on action against trafficking in human beings, Warsaw, 16.V.2005*. Retrieved from: https://rm.coe.int/16800d3812

Fineman, M. (2008). The vulnerable subject: Anchoring equality in the human condition. *Yale Journal of Law and Feminism, 20*(1), 1–23.

Fineman, M. (2009). Involving images of gender and equality: A feminist journey. *New England Law Review, 43*(3), 101–123.

Fineman, M. (2010). *The international law of human trafficking*. Cambridge, UK: University Press Cambridge.

Fineman, M. (2016). *Vulnerability. Reflections on a new ethical foundation for law and politics*. London: Taylor & Francis.

Gallagher, A. (2010). *The international law of human trafficking*. Cambridge, UK: University Press Cambridge.

Gallagher, A. (2012). *Issue paper on abuse of position of vulnerability and other "means" within of definition of trafficking in persons*. Vienna, Austria: UNODC.

Gallagher, A. (2015). *The concept of exploitation in the trafficking in persons protocol*. Vienna, Austria: UNODC.

Gallagher, A., & McAdam, M. (2017). Abuse of a position of vulnerability within the definition of trafficking persons. In R. Piotrowicz, C. Rijken, & B. Ulh (Eds.), *Handbook Human Trafficking* (pp. 185–198). London: Routledge.

Mackenzie, C., Rogers, W., & Dodds, S. (2014). *Vulnerability: New essays in ethics and feminist philosophy*. Oxford, UK: Oxford University Press.

Ministero della Giustizia. (2015). *Direzione generale di statistica e analisi organizzativa. La tratta degli esseri umani*. Retrieved from https://webstat.giustizia.it/Analisi%20e%20ricerche/Rapporto%20DgStat%20sulla%20tratta%20degli%20esseri%20umani.pdf

Nussbaum, M. (2011). *Creating capabilities: The human development approach*. Cambridge, MA: The Belknap Press of Harvard University Press.

OIM. (2017). La tratta di esseri umani attraverso la rotta del Mediterraneo centrale: dati, storie e informazioni raccolte dall'Organizzazione Internazionale per le migrazioni. Retrieved from https://italy.iom.int/sites/default/files/news-documents/RAPPORTO_OIM_Vittime_di_tratta_0.pdf

Pascoal, R. (2017). The analysis of the concept of vulnerability on the international legal framework on human trade. *Revista Debater a Europa, 17*(99), 97–114.

Penedo, R., & Wrabetz, J. (2015). Trafficking in human beings in time and space. A socioecological perspective. In M. J. Guia (Ed.), *The illegal business of human trafficking* (pp. 1–19). Cham, Switzerland: Springer Nature Switzerland.

Razack, S., Smith, M., & Thobani, S. (2011). *States of race: Critical race feminism for the 21st century*. Toronto, ON: Between the Lines.

Ricoeur, P. (2007). *Le juste*. Paris, France: Esprit.

Save the Children. (2019). *Piccoli schiavi invisibili 2019. Rapporto sui minori vittime di tratta e grave sfruttamento.* IX edizione. Retrieved from https://s3.savethechildren.it/public/files/uploads/pubblicazioni/piccoli-schiavi-invisibili-2019_0.pdf

Schütz, A. (1956). *Reflections on the problem of relevance*. New Haven, CT/London: Yale University Press.

Spivak, G. C. (1990). *The post-colonial critic: Interviews, strategies, dialogues*. London: Routledge.

UNODC. (2018). *The global report on trafficking in persons*. Vienna. Retrieved from https://www.unodc.org/documents/data-and-analysis/glotip/2018/GLOTiP_2018_BOOK_web_small.pdf. 20 Apr 2019.

UNODC, UNGIFT. (2008). *An introduction to human trafficking: Vulnerability, impact and action. Background paper.* Vienna. Retrieved from https://www.unodc.org/documents/human-trafficking/An_Introduction_to_Human_Trafficking_-_Background_Paper.pdf. 20 Apr 2019.

RULINGS Regarding Human Trafficking Passed by the Rumanian Supreme Court

Decizia nr. 131/RC/2016 Şedinţa publică din data de 19 aprilie 2016, https://www.scj.ro/1093/Detalii-jurisprudenta?customQuery%5B0%5D.Key=id&customQuery%5B0%5D.Value=130996, 21/03/2019.

Decizia nr. 134/A/2018 Şedinţa publică din data de 29 mai 2018, https://www.scj.ro/1093/Detalii-jurisprudenta?customQuery%5B0%5D.Key=id&customQuery%5B0%5D.Value=145672, 20/03/2019.

Decizia nr. 162/RC/2016 Şedinţa publică din data de 05 mai 2016, https://www.scj.ro/1093/Detalii-jurisprudenta?customQuery%5B0%5D.Key=id&customQuery%5B0%5D.Value=134631, 21/03/2019.

Decizia nr. 193/RC/2017 Şedinţa publică din data de 11 mai 2017, https://www.scj.ro/1093/Detalii-jurisprudenta?customQuery%5B0%5D.Key=id&customQuery%5B0%5D.Value=145706, 20/03/2019.

Decizia nr. 331/RC/2017, Şedinţa publică din 14 septembrie 2017, https://www.scj.ro/1093/Detalii-jurisprudenta?customQuery%5B0%5D.Key=id&customQuery%5B0%5D.Value=140968, 21/03/2019.

R O M Â N I A ÎNALTA CURTE DE CASAŢIE ŞI JUSTIŢIE. Secţia Penală.

RULINGS Regarding Human Trafficking Passed by the Italian Supreme Court

Cassazione penale – Sezione III, *Sentenza n. 32322* (ud. 05/02/2015, dep. 23/07/2015), in https://dejure.it/#/ricerca/giurisprudenza_documento?idDatabank=3&idDocMaster=4711203&idUnitaDoc=0&nVigUnitaDoc=1&isCorrelazioniSearch=true, 10/06/2019.

Cassazione penale – Sezione V, *Sentenza n. 5703* (ud. 22-10-2018, dep. 05-02-2019), in https://dejure.it/#/ricerca/giurisprudenza_documento?idDatabank=3&idDocMaster=7820064&idUnitaDoc=0&nVigUnitaDoc=1&docIdx=1&semantica=0&isPdf=false&fromSearch=true&isCorrelazioniSearch=false

Cassazione penale –Sezione V, *Sentenza n. 4275* (ud. 16/05/2017, dep. 19/09/2017), in https://dejure.it/#/ricerca/giurisprudenza_documento?idDatabank=3&idDocMaster=6270617&idUnitaDoc=0&nVigUnitaDoc=1&isCorrelazioniSearch=true, 11/06/2019.

Cassazione penale – Sezione V, *Sentenza n. 8545* (ud. 16/11/2018, dep. 27/02/2019), in https://dejure.it/#/ricerca/giurisprudenza_documento?idDatabank=3&idDocMaster=7852026&idUnitaDoc=0&nVigUnitaDoc=1&docIdx=1&semantica=0&isPdf=false&fromSearch=true&isCorrelazioniSearch=false

Cassazione penale – Sezione V, *Sentenza n. 34403* (ud. 03-06-2015, dep. 06-08-2015), in https://dejure.it/#/ricerca/giurisprudenza_documento?idDatabank=3&idDocMaster=4718848&idUnitaDoc=0&nVigUnitaDoc=1&docIdx=4&semantica=0&isPdf=false&fromSearch=true&isCorrelazioniSearch=false

Chapter 4
Nostalgia and Proximity Violence: Daily Life and Regressive *Mestizament*

4.1 Introduction

The changed human geography of the cities of "southern Europe" (Cassano, 1996) – where immigrants who have arrived some time ago and refugees–asylum seekers awaiting residential permits mingle with the inhabitants of the most popular neighbourhoods – is also reflected in the possible hybridization of different cultural representations, at times, completely different relational dynamics.

Numerous sociological studies and a broad variety of case studies highlight how migrants, conceived as people (with their uniqueness, concreteness, culture, relationality) and not as individuals (abstract and fungible), are often conditioned by the social systems with which they enter into contact without however having been being determined by them. A form of reluctance ascribable to sedimented cultural factors constituting immigrants' identitarian backgrounds prevents them from making the culture of the host country their own. The society of Mediterranean Europe contains a wide range of micro-worlds which have created segmented rapports while each fragment has maintained its own intrinsic characteristics. Contact occurs regardless of attempts made to foster integration because they are oriented mainly towards the instrumental pursuit of the (few) advantages – economic or otherwise practical – the host communities offer. This integration of the migrant is often strategic and surface. Furthermore, procedures involved do not concern the migrants only but, to some extent, the indigenous population too. The creation of opportunities for exchange and the promotion of intercultural knowledge are among the practices that the Italian SPRAR system provides for and imposes upon operators involved in reception. In the case of migrants who have settled in southern Italian cities and have been residents for a longer period than newcomers, relations with the original population are usually aimed at solving problems shared by all – work or housing, cohabitation in condominiums or neighbourhoods, etc. In actual fact, the practical interest shown by the migrant or migrant family corresponds to the equally

I. Bartholini, *The Trap of Proximity Violence*,
https://doi.org/10.1007/978-3-030-52451-7_4

practical interest of the native individual or family of the neighbourhood. So, if natives and immigrants find themselves interacting to solve problems of common interest in the same apartment building, workplace, or compulsory school attended by their children, the same cannot be said when it comes to behaviour related to the private sphere and the models cultural to which they refer. Therefore, if numerous studies reiterate the reluctance or slowness of the migrant population to prove reactive when it comes to the cultures of the host countries, the propensity of autochthonous peoples to mingle has been explored very little as yet. There has not been sufficient investigation of the incidence of conditionality regarding the opposite case, that is, the extent to which migrants contribute to changing the behaviour and points of view of the members of the host societies and communities. It is possible to hypothesize that under certain conditions the opposite effect is reached, that is, that representations of violence against women, proximity violence in particular, are subverted thanks to their specular interpretation by the autochthonous populations precisely by virtue of the "demonstration" provided by migrant groups.

Since migrants do not belong to some abstract category, they too, like the autochthonous people, should also be considered by age, group, profession, and, above all, gender. The latter is one of the elements most symptomatic of the entire structured and structuring migration process. This is why reciprocal subjectivities have been observed in one of the lowest-income neighbourhoods of Palermo where migration has produced the greatest impact and revealed the contradictory nature of procedural, dynamics involved. This inquiry presupposed an ex-ante understanding of processes of migration and their outcomes within that very neighbourhood while taking into account forms of *engendering migration* (Abbatecola & Bimbi, 2013) by carrying out a differential comparison between women and men as well as the selection of an all-female sample. In this sense, we started from the assumption that by retracing the individual trajectories (Freedman, 2015) generated by socialization within a network of hospitality provided by the county of arrival, meant initially, as explained in chapter two of this volume, establishing, from the beginning, the effects that the structures of gender, space and time both concrete and imaginary experienced by migrant women, might have had upon them within their home environments, during transit and upon arrival.

The project also explores and reflects on the effects that the habits and practices of immigrant women, informed by values of *shame and honour*, have on how they are perceived by some Palermitan women in relation to their own roles and identity. At a first glance, migrant and indigenous women might seem to find themselves at the antipodes: the former submissive, often victims of violence, the former fully engaged in a process of advanced emancipation, accompanied by a renewed kind of humanism founded on the principle that the worth of a human could not be reduced to differences of gender, class, social group, or economic interest. Apparently, in actual fact, the immigrant, like every other person, becomes, at least in part, the architect of the reality surrounding her, bearing witness to her own culture, to the active and passive practices of resistance externalized through their customs. The effect upon the autochthonous women may take the form of refusal of the cultural and social behaviour and models of conduct the immigrants bear, but it may, under certain conditions, induce them to question their own.

The hypothesis we embraced is that there is a mechanism which tends to reverse the effects and achievements of women's empowerment movements. Violence, as an effect of the mestizament between migrant and Euro-Mediterranean cultures, has been investigated very little within a general underestimation of how much the heritage of our patriarchate may re-emerge reinvigorated precisely due to the material and symbolic impact of contemporary migration. It is possible to assume that one of the least desirable outcomes of the encounter between migrant and indigenous cultures is a sort of regressive mestizament, evident above all in the *Lebenswelt* of social groups culturally less equipped who live in close contact with the newcomers in the popular neighbourhoods of the urban areas.

A few but significant other studies have intercepted this risk: a recent review, carried out at European level, reveals how a small but significant proportion of respondents (young people and victims included) tends to justify some violent behaviour against women, highlighting attitudes of widespread general acceptance and tolerance regarding it (Gracia & Lila, 2015). The data provided by the 2014 Istat survey and the results of previous Urban Report (Basaglia, Lotti, Misiti, & Tola, 2007) also reveal the existence and persistence in Italy of value systems and social constructs that include levels of acceptance of violence even by those who have experienced it.

The hypothesis that this chapter endeavoured to verify was how and to what extent migratory processes contributed to the reappearance or reinvigoration of the "honour-and-shame" paradigm (Bartholini, 2016; Giordano, 1994; Peristiany, 1965; Peristiany & Pitt-Rivers, 1991), within dynamics relating to the material and symbolic organization of gender relations, within social contexts of migrant hospitality. It also sought to show how these factors affect, indirectly, perceptions and evaluations of indigenous groups of the images conveyed by migrants.

4.2 Economic Links and Behavioural Consequences

This study limits its area of investigation to one of Palermo's oldest and most popular districts – *Ballarò* – to give an account of the interpretation provided by Palermitan women regarding the gender discrimination suffered by migrant women in their daily lives and their relationships with their partners, brothers, and fellow countrymen.

Furthermore, it also aimed at pondering on the possibility that the evaluations they themselves provide regarding why they willingly accepted practices of segregation based on *male domination*, may influence the local women, even raise doubts regarding the "goodness" of their codes of behaviour compared to those of the foreign women living in the same area of Palermo. From this angle, the neighbourhood where the research was carried out acted as an arena of meaning and the field within which negotiations between indigenous and immigrant women take place regarding reciprocal representations and their subsequent positions. There were many indicators which we might have considered, but for our case study we focused on two elements that characterize the neighbourhood: income as a measure of well-being and education as an indicator of human development. In the first case, income, there is substantial homogeneity between the incomes of the autochthonous and migrant populations, a per capita homogeneity lower than 300 euros a month which drops to 268 if the female population is taken into consideration. If we consider the levels of education and the duration of school attendance of the inhabitants of the neighbourhood, the average time span is 7 years and 1 month, lower than the time foreseen in Italy for compulsory schooling. When it comes to migrant women living in the neighbourhood the average time spent in education falls to 5 years and 2 months. Furthermore, in this district, as in the peripheral neighbourhoods of many parts of southern Italy, the situation remains constantly critical because of the scarce application of policies aimed at human development in general in terms of investments in education or health; even more so when it comes to the application to woman of equal-opportunity policies as a substantive right whereby men and women should be provided with identical chances of education. The economic elements that prevent human development, according to the *capability approach*, highlights if applied to the *Ballarò* district, the impossibility of isolating the economic issue from other fundamental aspects of the life of each individual. The development of each person – man or woman – is both a condition and consequence of economic development, of the relationship between commodities and capabilities (Nussbaum, 2000; Sen, 1999, 2007) which has an impact on the problem of equality between people. The distribution of economic resources among citizens should take place by a *trickle-down* chain effect capable of reaching those who are at the bottom of the hierarchical ladder. The *Ballarò* neighbourhood, with its high unemployment rate and where undeclared work is almost the only source of employment, finds in the help provided by the social services a necessary contribution to daily survival. This is how women are driven into the poverty trap which becomes even more suffocating when they have children to support and find themselves alone because of being divorced or separated de facto. In these peculiar conditions, the women of the popular neighbourhoods endure double poverty as women and as mothers. It then happens that the relationship between women's emancipation that has permitted women to work outside the home is a practical failure precisely when it comes to social groups where unemployment among the least competent is most rampant. These are female breadwinners who have no chance of developing their skills and whose social status makes them visible in their individual contexts. In addition to this, there exists a situational vulnerability due to marital abandonment, failed marriages, divorces, separations or, on the contrary, due to forced cohabitation dictated by economic need. In both cases, these women who experience double poverty – economic and social – and double responsibility – are often those forced to take care of themselves and their children without the help of a partner due to contextual (like unemployment) and situational (private) problems, who observe with some curiosity and a certain amazement the type of migrant woman who in the *Ballarò* district reveals her modesty and a certain private security – that of having a father or husband willing to provide their basic family needs.

4.3 Violence and Retrospective Interpretation of Violence

Johan Galtung (1969) in the article "Violence, Peace, and Peace Research" identified three core components of violence: direct, structural, and cultural.

At the upmost tip stands the direct manifestation of a personal form of injustice likely traceable to concrete subjects. By way of contrast, structural violence is an indirect process of exploitation and marginalization that is not always perceived by the entire community. Incorporated amid the deeper layers of the triangle lies cultural violence, the process through which violence comes to be seen as natural and legitimate.

Representations of Violence according to Galtung

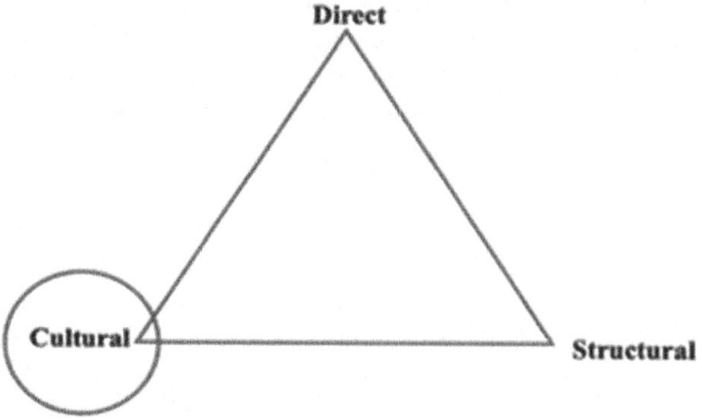

Just as the migrant women (Aziza, Folucke, and Ghana) through their accounts have acknowledged direct violence along with its possible categories clearly, even more so the Palermitan women interviewed have represented direct immediately recognizable aspects of violence. The problem and its viscous connections, on the other hand, concern the ability/possibility of recognizing the contextual and cultural dynamics of violence. In attempting to unravel the nodes of influence existing between "exotic" and "native" practices and representations, the researcher clearly needs to analyse the effects of antithetical cultural thrusts impacting upon an opaque area with uncertain borders. The first, modernist, still rooted in the patriarchal paradigm, expressed primarily through gender relations based on control over women, seems to be represented by migrant women in particular. The other although it cannot be defined post-modern may be considered intersectional and, by aiming to consider some of the subordinate axes experienced by women simultaneously, underlines the need to distinguish between differences and consider the specific vulnerability of each woman also on the basis of the processes of resistance set in motion in each specific situation.

In the following pages we aim at highlighting some of the roles found in gender dynamics, by shedding light on processes of resistance set up by migrant women and reflected in the Palermitan women's perception of who share some socializing circumstances with them.

The description of the viscous links between the vulnerability (Kirby, 2006) and resistance (Butler, Gambetti, & Sabsay, 2016; Bracke, 2016) of migrant women submitted to a patriarchal culture or victims of violence, is important when seeking to pursue a line which is also and above all practical when it comes to male domination, to how it is exercised through and in relations between subjects, in order to highlight the effects that these links have within broader spheres of sociality. They are expressed both during incorporation into the *habitus* and in the mental setup of victims and perpetrators as actions and interactions. Resistance as a response by migrant women to proximity violence, intended as the most "intimate and difficult to eradicate" (Bartholini, 2016) form of gender-based violence, confirms the presence of a patriarchal culture that impresses, when it does not fascinate the autochthonous women themselves.

The background of this research was that culture laboratories set up in the *Ballarò* district, whose native population lives in close contact with the migrant and asylum-seeking population. Their relationships unfold, beyond the family (Dahlberg, Dahlberg, & Nyström, 2008), in a context where they share many daily actions with the immigrant women of the neighbourhood, thus broadening their mutual panorama of reference.

This chapter presents, within a multi-year participant observation project, the results of research involving six focus groups where 30 Palermitan women took part in numerically smaller groups. They shared with the first- and second-generation African women of the *Ballarò* district, a daily life comprising actions and situations which create bonds of sociality attributable to daily life like shopping at the market or in the same local shops, going to the school, meetings their children's, management of the cleaning roster of the condominiums where they reside, etc.

Thirty women, eight of whom separated de facto, who, as neighbours belonging to the district or direct acquaintances of the foreign women interviewed in Chap. 2, were in some way involuntary spectators of the roles played by the former. These testimonies aimed at verifying, – although, at first glance, this undertaking was scientifically "audacious" – whether the patterns of conduct and behaviour of migrant women might have some influence on Palermitan women belonging to a cultural milieu which appeared to have freed itself from the patriarchy upon which gender relations had long been based within the environment of reference.

All this for the purpose of verifying whether the issue of female subordination and exploitation, attributable to cultural models at the basis of the socialization processes experienced in the countries of origin by migrant women, once reproduced in the host countries, might influence broader social circles and contribute to a re-proposal and partial re-legitimization of paradigms of the past based on the "honour-and-shame" conceptual dyad. So, if it were possible to highlight some aspects of a regressive mestizament between the segregationist cultures of the newcomers from the African continent – Cameroon, Tanzania, Zimbabwe, Congo, Nigeria, South Sudan, etc. – and those of the autochthonous women living in the district of Palermo where the research project was conducted.

4.4 The Research

Often, a considerable amount of knowledge regarding the original background of the interviewees helps the researcher to maintain a neutral approach, thus avoiding potential "pollution" of the topic of the research. This theoretical approach proves particularly advantageous when it comes to exploring behaviour and action involved in interaction (De Wal, 1992), while also preventing a priori emphases capable of influencing the results of research at different levels.

In the qualitative methodology used in this research, the participant observation carried out before and during the non-directive interviews allowed for better interaction between the researcher and the women interviewed (Bonner & Tolhurst, 2002). The basic aim of the interviews at the very heart of the research consisted in accessing the "*perspective of the subjects studied*" (Corbetta, 2015: 70), that is, in interpreting their representations of the world and the reasons attributed to their actions. The latter are fundamental when seeking to identify the elements ascribable to patriarchy and legitimization of the production and reproduction of specific representations.

The sample of Palermitan women comprised women with children – married (17), cohabiting (5), or separated (8), with a poor level of education. After compulsory schooling, they had preferred to learn a trade (as a hairdresser, cook, seamstress, etc.), so they told us, or had chosen not to continue their studies anyway; they did not work outside the home, except occasionally as charwomen, carers, street vendors, and were aged between 25 and 44.

They shared some aspects of daily life with the migrant women like shopping at the market or waiting for their children outside of the school or cleaning the buildings in which they lived.

Among the research participants four were street vendors (two had fruit and vegetable stalls, one sold fish, one women's clothing) in the local market also called *Ballarò*, 6 were carers, 18 unemployed, 2 declared to work "illegally". In addition, 21 of them had children who attended classes with the immigrant children while 14 of them lived in apartment buildings where migrant families lived too. All of them were residents of the *Ballarò* district.

The aim of the four focus groups was to highlight forms of cross-contamination between cultures and the intersections where proximity violence, marred by exoticism, if attributed to a different culture, was tolerated. This mixture may also be interpreted through the lens of a *capability approach* which takes into consideration the process which allows one to act in relation to peoples' actual possibilities and opportunities, taking into account the conditions in which they live and how much a failure to develop personal resources may favour a different interpretation of what would be considered differently in other conditions/situations.

A second objective was to evaluate, precisely by virtue of the potential empowerment acquired by the women interviewed, the interpretation they provided of the violence of proximity of which migrant women are bearers. Individual empowerment is a process that we researchers intended as progress among the women of the neighbourhood and considered ex ante as that particular process whereby individuals acquire skills, increase their ability to take active control their own lives and develop critical awareness of their social, political, organizational, and cultural environment (Zimmerman, 2000).

The aim of the focus groups was to bring to the surface positions that the participants assumed with respect to the behaviour patterns manifested by migrant women with a view to highlighting their perception of them (Råheim et al., 2016) and using them as a mirror to their own. By observing the "Other women" they highlighted how the segregation or violence suffered by immigrant women produced a distinctly different interpretation of what the Palermitan women beheld as indirect witnesses.

> *I see them every day, the two Muslims who live right here with their children and husband, we say hello, often buy from me and talk ... more than talk we understand each other, regarding the price of vegetables, what they would like to find and what there is in their markets that cannot be found here. Sometimes I ask them for information about how they cook mutton or ... if they make couscous, that's all. I'm curious, I'd like to talk about something else. For example, I would like to know if their magic rituals are really effective ... but they are very "tight lipped" ....* (Giovanna, 39 years old street vendor)

> *She goes out accompanied, is twenty and already has a child but when other Muslims come out, they walk in front of her and she behind ... she is never alone.* (Vincenza, 36 years old, lives in a building where immigrant families live too)

> *They always go out in groups, at least 3 or 4, to go to the mosque. It would be impossible for a man from this neighbourhood to stop them and even have a chat.* (Milena, 36, living in the neighbourhood)

> *They are like us, but older than us in their heads although younger in age. A few days ago, my daughter celebrated her birthday. She celebrated it at home, nothing special ... Sara wanted to know if there would be boys and especially older boys, because in that case her daughter would not even ask her father's permission. I say ... the daughter is 12, not 4 years old ... permission to come to my house?!* (Patrizia, 33, mother of a schoolmate of a migrant girl).

> *They have three children, two boys and one girl. The boys play on the street, I have never seen the girl alone. She goes out only with her mother.* (Francesca, 41 years old, a neighbour)

> *They told me that when she went to the Cervello hospital to give birth, she absolutely refused being cut. She was infibulated - they told me - and the social worker who accompanied her did not know how to convince her. She was infibulated and since here, after giving birth, the doctors do not perform these practices, they would not have - let's say - mended her; she did not want to give birth. She cried out in pain but didn't want to be cut. In the end, the doctor carried out a caesarean section ... the only way to save mother and child ... by cesarean, even if it wouldn't have been necessary. Madness. But did she really want to die?* (Giuseppina, 44, social worker at a SPRAR)

> *When I see them at school, all covered and I think of the mothers of some of our children, who go to get their children to be looked at, I say that they are better.* (Maria, 33 years old, mother of a schoolmate of a migrant)

Yes, for my son I would like a Moroccan or Tunisian wife, because you can see they are ladies; they have the same colour skin as us skin and yet they are calmer, more mature than their age, they care more about the family. They do not cheat on their husbands; my son could have a more peaceful life, his father would not worry, because he sees them – here – a hundred times better... much better ... (Francesca, 41 years old, neighbour)

I have been married twice but am alone again. I had three children with the first husband and one with the second. They live upstairs. Sometimes I hear the husband shouting, I hear her cry. But sometimes I even hear her sing. You see, maybe ... I'm not saying it's good to get beaten but maybe I, if I had been less nervous, if I had counted to ten before slamming the doors and leaving, I would still have a husband. You see, back then I thought I was "an expert", that I would not yield ... instead what have I achieved? (Rosaria, 45 years old, neighbour)

Yes, she wears a veil ... always, yet she does not lose her temper, always obeys her husband, cooks, oh how much she cooks while her daughter tidies the house up... I never see her standing still ... but I don't even see her angry ... never ... she never gets angry ... well for her. (Francesca, 41 years old, neighbour)

I tell you a house. It is true that Fathima does not leave the house without her children or her husband, and wears a veil, and I have never seen her knees. But if she goes to the market, she tells her husband what she wants to buy and he pays. I used to wear short skirts but my husband had no money and worked only occasionally. I, wearing short skirts have been going to clean the stairs for years. Before I liked it, I felt I was being looked at, then I thought that if my husband cared about my thighs, he wouldn't have allowed me to expose them. (Gessica, 29 years old, charlady)

Yes, I know, her patch is near the station, but she is the one who brings the money home for everyone. For her son and for that paracite of a Michele who sleeps all day. No, I wouldn't. I would have thrown him out of the house. already But I admire her for what she does, for the sacrifices she makes. Yes, she knows the word love ... even if she sells herself ... because it sells herself to make the other two feel good. (Vincenza, 35 years old, neighbour)

The excerpts quoted here describe a gradual process of acceptance and justification of the patriarchal dynamics of segregation and proximity violence, as well as exploitation, which the Palermitan women who participated in the focus groups associate with migrant women. It emerged from the fieldwork that migrant women are defined in terms of country of birth, ethnicization, gender, and tend to be associated with specific behaviour viewed almost favourably by the native women of the neighbourhood. The vulnerability and resistance of the foreign women is considered positively by the native women interviewed, even when their relationships are evaluated negatively (think, for example, of Vincenza's testimony full of admiration for the prostitute who sacrifices herself for the people in her care). The respect, albeit veiled by irony, which transpires from the opinions expressed by the women of *Ballarò* means that not only gender segregation, but even violence – when it is proximal – that is, undergone within intimate or emotional ties, is contextually justified and becomes a source of respect and admiration. In addition, more than one testimony refers to how economic resources are shared within the migrant family despite the discrimination suffered by the female partner. The kind of empowerment expressed is negative.

Empowerment – except in Freire (1975) – refers precisely to that kind of awareness (through information) and to concrete and real capacity ability to rebel against oppressors and impose, instead, situation favourable to the individual who rebels. It is precisely the empowerment process, as that kind of social action whereby people, organizations, and communities take change of their own lives to improve gender equality and quality of life (Zimmerman, 2000), seems not to have achieved the desired effects.

It is also possible to catch glimpses of embryonic forms of emulation of those very same women who have succeeded in transforming their vulnerability into resistance without breaches, in the wake of a tradition which, though remote from the everyday life of the Palermitan women, seems, however, to be appreciated with some nostalgia. The violence suffered, sometimes exhibited, by the migrant women, as a mark of resistance on their part, becomes a deforming mirror where love and endurance become mingled in the eyes of the Palermitan women, with love tout court. This is a romantic kind of love imbued with "belonging", despite the fact that romantic love has always been unbalanced from the point of view of gender, as a result of (historical-cultural) conditioning, and actually remains unbalanced from the point of view of power, too. Far too often "dreams of romantic love have pushed women into domestic submission" (Giddens, 1992: 71). And, as Bell Hooks writes, "in our country, masses of people are affected by violence, but they insist on not linking this violence to patriarchal thought or male domination" (2016: 83).

This negative symbolic coefficient, which often characterizes African women, now seems to re-manifest itself in some of the attitudes of the autochthonous women as a consequence of mestizament between the cultures of migrants and natives, in the negotiation of symbolic or material goods that constantly reshape the internal logic and boundaries of exchange. The focus groups conducted with the women of Palermo permitted the emergence of expressions of respect, even of admiration for the "shame-and-honour" behavioural patterns, postures, and attitudes (Peristiany, 1965), of African women living in the neighbourhood. The interviewees remembered that these patterns were typical of their grandmothers and relatives from a more distant past. These memories of the past were judged positively by them especially when it came to the marital stability of which African women are representatives. Nostalgia, therefore, of a past that seemed to provide greater certainty than a present where emancipation has made the interviewees more vulnerable with respect to both their private and social lives. When assessing the "attitudes" of immigrant women, participants in the focus groups remarked how decision-making, the result of previous battles which made them potentially emancipated women and female breadwinners, has done nothing to bridge the *gender equity gender equality* gap. While the latter refers to an equal enjoyment of resources by men and women and to equivalence of *outcome,* regardless of differences in situation and context, *gender equity* refers to fairness between men and women, redistribution of power and resources according to the situation in which everyone lives regardless of whether the subject is a woman or man. The testimonies – as well as the statistical data – revealed that because there had been substantial difficulty in making gender equity as foreseen by the law comply with gender equity de facto in the cases of the women interviewed, this led them to re-evaluate the marital and family strategies observed in the migrant women of the *Ballarò* district.

The testimonies brought to light the direct relationship between the framework of "exotic" representations of gender relations and a general regression towards a revival of forms of patriarchy. The disturbing aspect of this stage of the research is that respect and nostalgia for the gender dynamics of the past denote a regressive cultural effect of mestizament on local women who, while recognizing the negative effects of gender segregation, remain influenced by it, sometimes, even fascinated. It reveals a re-emergence, thanks to the "devotional" models of subordination to the male represented by the migrant woman in exchange for economic tranquillity, of traces of patriarchalism nostalgically recalled by the Sicilian women who, although backed by modest arguments, encourage a return to past models where vulnerability and resistance converged in the feminine.

4.5 Conclusions

What we feel emerges at the end of this research is how "We are very different, but we are also manifestly similar. So, what (complex) social arrangements derive from these similarities and differences?" (Walzer, 2007). An increasing number of international studies and reports reveal a general process of justification of the violence attributed to specific groups (Bograd, 1999; Flood & Pease 2009; Gracia & Lila, 2015) by autochthonous groups. The representations of gender segregation and interpretations of the phenomenon do not pertain, however, to a currently enrolled, single interpretative paradigm but are themselves the product of a hybrid combination of paradigms and different cultural tensions often diachronic and confused.

Moreover:

1. The intersectional (Carastathis, 2016; Crenshaw, 1991) approach teaches us that there are interlocking oppressions which go beyond a dichotomous understanding of the oppositional differences (Collins, 1986: 20).
2. The feminist theory (Collins, 1986; Haraway, 2004; Harding, 1991, 2004) teaches us that "knowledge is socially situated; marginalized groups are socially situated in ways that make it more possible for them to be aware of things and ask questions than it is for the non-marginalized; research, particularly that focused on power relations, should begin with the lives of the marginalized" (Harding, 2007: 352–355). Intersectional analysis helps us to understand interlocking oppressions (Campbell, 2015).

The testimonies of 30 women of Palermitan origin, all residing in the *Ballarò* district of the city, show how much some of the behaviour patterns of the migrant women interviewed influence the attitudes and behavioural codes of those who reside within the same social spheres as them. And this, whether they are hosted in reception centres, or now live permanently in the multiracial neighbourhoods of the city suburbs of western Sicily. Moreover, as highlighted in Chap. 2, the testimonies collected through the interviews administered to the sample of migrant women not only favoured the collection of a large repertoire of cases of proximity and gender violence, of segregation, but also they allowed us to analyse the dynamics of vulnerability and resistance involving acceptance of relationships on their part. The findings highlighted the possible viscous effects that their behaviour produces in the daily life of those who, although not part of their family networks, share aspects of sociality with them or become indirect spectators of their daily lives. Women – immigrant and autochthonous – much more than men, find themselves participating in a daily life routine made of shopping at the market, housework, and caring for their children, which in fact breaks down some of the apparent cultural barriers. And this would seem to confirm the Bourdieusian thesis whereby "whatever their position in the social sphere, women have in common the fact of being separated from men by a negative symbolic coefficient which, like the colour of the skin for blacks, is a sign of membership of a group to be discriminated and therefore has a negative effect on everything they are and do" (Bourdieu, 1998: 100).

From this point of view, the emotional structures of the foreign women interviewed seem completely separate from the economic logic of their partners, and are closely linked to the way in which a patriarchal culture continues to interpret shame as a producer of order of their reality is male dominion which appears unsurpassed and unreformable precisely because it is exercised through proxemic violence.

The representation of these asymmetric balances with roots in gender segregation, however, is found in the native women in a mixture of attraction and repulsion revealing regressive mestizament, a shift backwards of *their* order of things towards a past which appears partially idealized and expurged of segregation which it used to contain. This regressive mestizament is one of the unexpected effects of the traps of violence. According to the results of this survey, it is a trap into which those women who have not been supported in the context emancipation fall. Living in a poor neighbourhood has not allowed them to achieve real and total emancipation.

As Bimbi wrote recently, "the Mediterranean area has interpreted the honour-and-shame paradigm" (ibidem: 46) as well as male–female relations. And although it seems to constitute an anachronistic residue of a postmodern type of society, it continues to spread through groups of newcomers, and generally favours reverberations of proximal violence.

The paradigm of honour is a stain which has distinguished a large part of European-Mediterranean cultures and legitimized a behavioural code which has been openly opposed only since the 1970s, after the Sicilian Franca Viola's "refusal" to legitimize rape by a reparatory marriage, seems to be raising its head again today. Proof of this are the data from the statistics that constantly record increases in cases of gender-based violence and feminicides in Italy and those from the confessions and declarations made by the perpetrators of these acts.

On the other hand, the entry of women from Africa, victims of sexual exploitation, proposes in actual fact the possibility of coercive use of women's bodies, especially when "already violated", already "abused" during the journey to the Mediterranean coasts. On the other hand, the testimonies of the immigrant women gathered here have highlighted the presence of a widespread submission of women within traditional relationship dynamics, based on specific religious and cultural models. These also end up by proposing a "local" patriarchalism.

To separate the discourse on proximity violence undergone by the sample of immigrant women interviewed from the cultural representations which justify it, as well as the processes of vulnerability and resistance implemented, would mean separating it from possible interpretations that "naturalize" it, which would produce a sort of "racialization" of migrants (Crenshaw, 1991; Razack, 2011).

A common aspect of the research, which rotates around the gender segregation and patriarchalism exhibited by the newcomers, is that for the majority of the women interviewed, proximity violence is permitted, tolerated, and justified within a traditional view of the couple or may be due to emotional dependence defining their extended vulnerability (Bartholini, 2013, 2015; Bimbi, 2015). From this angle, patriarchalism is not only an interpretative category of violence referring to the economic, cultural, or religious peculiarities of the actors, but finds its epistemic characterization in that violence that is perpetrated against victims by a person or persons close to them, both in the case of Ghana's abuse-ridden journey, that of Foluke's exploitation as a prostitute, and the forced marriage of Aziza, where an "intimate" perpetrator, a neighbour is legitimized by the law and tradition. The conduct of the interviewees shows that violence is considered a problem only when it degenerates or/and the circle of perpetrators extends outside of the proximity relationship.

An unexpected aspect, however, is in the very scope of what we have identified as the dawn of a regressive kind of mestizament, the effects of which were characterized by a number of different nuances due precisely to the considerations of the autochthonous women who assessed the behaviour and daily actions of women immigrants belonging to their district positively. Having recorded, during the focus groups involving the Palermitan women living in the *Ballarò* district, attitudes marked by respect for segregationist practices to which African women were subjected and, having registered opinions and observations cloaked in nostalgia when dealing with family systems which appear, to the Sicilian women, as stable and solid, as regards both the division of roles within the families of the newcomers, and the moral aspects of marital fidelity, let us suppose that the contacts between them lead to some regression by the Palermo women interviewed. The same seem to confuse the logics of male domination with the modernist ones of indissoluble marriage and seem to neglect how African women find themselves within segregationist systems certainly not chosen by them. They also seem to evaluate the recent past of their mothers and grandmothers as a temporal reality undoubtedly more reassuring than what they are experiencing at present, and more similar to that of African immigrant women whom they meet every day. Some of the interviewees have openly stated that if their son married an African, he would be more likely to be shielded from the instability which characterizes contemporary couples.

Globalized migrations seem, therefore, to mark a social change based on two biases which highlight a more generally regressive kind of mestizament. The first is to have erroneously taken the end of male hegemony for granted and conceive the phenomenology of male violence against women in "our" world as pre-modern.

The second is that of representing Western culture as emancipated, leaving in the shade diversified reproductions of symbolic (Bourdieu, 1998) and real violence that exist in our reference environments.

The intersectional approach also highlighted how gender is necessary though not sufficient as a category to interpret dynamics and trajectories. These are influenced also by the differences that characterize each of the participants in the research, and each woman in general, incorporates (Crenshaw, 1991; Nixon & Humphreys, 2010), and which may be attributed to the level of schooling received by each woman and to the social class to which she belongs. Proximity violence suggests a wider field of analysis than that attributable purely to the phenomenology of gender-based violence; it points towards an intersection between frequently disparate social phenomena, an understanding of which permits us:

1. To note how the so-called *gender gap* persists both within and outside the family with effects deriving from social and cultural difficulties that favour the emergence of new dyscrasias regarding the distribution of tasks and the creation of roles.
2. To intercept sizeable transformations resulting from globalized migration and socio-cultural changes taking place in the post-patriarchal societies of Mediterranean Europe.

In this sense, these representations seem to revise, in the unsaid insinuating itself into the European-Mediterranean consciousness, the fascination of the centuries-old exercise of the power of man over women's bodies. The more these representations are socially tolerated, it seems, the more they conceal mechanisms that still need to be analysed. Here a "historical unconscious" which eludes the individual will and consciousness is at work. It is so deeply insinuated into the body and in the hereditary burden that the genders carry with them, that we cannot truly imagine that it can be changed by decree or by an act of the will.

Today, Mediterranean is a workshop where (without interruption) discordant, modernist, and post-modern behavioural patterns actually persist (Collins, 2008; Corradi, 2009). It is precisely this mix which makes any balance precarious and facilitates reaffirmation of violent conduct legitimized by sexist logic (Edwards, 1987; Garcia-Moreno, Jansen, Ellsberg, Heise, & Watts, 2006; Gillioz, De Puy, & Ducret, 2000) which appeared to have been relegated to the recent past. Virginia Wolf (1927) would have identified this precarious balance with a reproduction of *Macht*: regurgitations of male violence that emerge in everyday life, "matches struck unexpectedly in the dark".

Encounters between migrant and indigenous cultures are actually producing a *regressive mestizament.* This phenomenon is favoured by a lack of the development of commodities and services as well as by the aptitude of the autochthonous women of the culturally less equipped social groups who live in close contact with the newcomers to popular urban neighbourhoods. This mestizament emerges as an institutional form of violence impacting upon the nostalgic effects of the proximity violence of which migrant women are victims, turning it into a "veritable gilded cage".

References

Abbatecola, E., & Bimbi, F. (2013). Introduction. Engenderin migrations. *Mondi Migranti. Rivista di Studi di Studi e Ricerche sulle Migrazioni Internazionali, 3*, 31–47.

Bartholini, I. (2013). *Violenza di prossimità. La vittima, il carnefice, lo spettatore e il "grande occhio"*. Milan, Italy: FrancoAngeli.

Bartholini, I. (Ed.). (2015). *Violenza di genere e percorsi mediterranei. Voci, saperi, uscite*. Milan, Italy: Guerini e Associati.

Bartholini, I. (2016). Emancipazione pubblica privata. Tratteggi di una gender violence tardo moderna nell'incrociarsi di paradigmi atlantici e mediterranei. *Autonomie locali e servizio sociale, 2*(3), 56–81.

Basaglia, A., Lotti, M. R., Misiti, M., & Tola, V. (Ed.) (2007). Il silenzio e le parole. *Il rapporto nazionale Rete Antiviolenza fra le città Urban-Italia*. Dipartimento per i diritti e le pari opportunità Presidenza del Consiglio dei Ministri, Rome.

bell Hooks. (2016). Farla finita con la violenza. In S. Vaccaro (Ed.), *Violenza di genere. Saperi contro*. Milan, Italy: Mimesis.

Bimbi, F. (2015). Onore-e-vergogna. Il ritorno di un paradigma mediterraneo nel dibattito europeo. In I. Bartholini (Ed.), *Violenza di genere e percorsi mediterranei. Voci, saperi, uscite* (pp. 27–44). Milan, Italy: Guerini e Associati.

Bograd, F. (1999). Strengthening domestic violence theories: Intersections of race, class, sexual orientation, and gender. *Journal of Marital and Family Therapy, 25*, 275–289.

Bonner,·A., & Tolhurst, G. (2002). Insider-outsider perspectives of participant observation. *Nurse Researcher, 9*(4), 7–19.

Bourdieu, F. (1998). *La nomination masculine*. Paris, France: Edition di Seul.

Bracke, S. (2016). Bouncing back: Vulnerability and resistance in times of resilience. In J. Butler, Z. Gambetti, & L. Sabsay (Eds.), *Vulnerability and resistance* (pp. 52–75). Durham, NC: Duke University Press.

Butler, J., Gambetti, Z., & Sabsay, L. (2016). *Vulnerability in resistance*. Durham, NC: Duke University Press.

Campbell, M. (2015). CEDAW and women's intersecting identities: A pioneering new approach to intersectional discrimination. *Revista Di reito GV, 11*(2), 479–504.

Carastathis, A. (2016). *Intersectionality: Origins, contestations, horizons*. Lincoln, OR: University of Nebraska Press.

Cassano, F. (1996). *Il pensiero meridiano*. Rome, Italy/Bari, Italy: Laterza.

Collins, P. H. (1986). Learning from the outsider within: The sociological significance of black feminist thought. *Social Problems, 33*(6), 14–32.

Collins, R. (2008). *Violence. A micro-sociological theory*. Princeton, NJ: Princeton University Press.

Corbetta, P. (2015). *Metodologia e tecniche della ricerca sociale*. Bologna, Italy: Il Mulino.

Corradi, C. (2009). *Sociologia della violenza. Modernità, identità, potere*. Rome, Italy: Meltemi.

Crenshaw, K. (1991). Mapping: Intersectionality, identity politics and violence against women of colour. *Standford Law Review, 43*, 124–129.

Dahlberg, K., Dahlberg, H., & Nyström, M. (2008). *Reflective lifeworld research*. Lund, Sweden: Studentlitteratur.

De Wal, F. (1992). Intentional deception in primates. *Evolutionary Anthropology, 1*(3), 86–92.

Edwards, E. (1987). Male violence in feminist theory: An analysis of the changing conceptions of sex/gender violence and male dominance. In J. Hanmer & M. Maynard (Eds.), *Women, violence and social control. Explorations in sociology*. London: Macmillan.

Flood, M., & Pease, B. (2009). Factors influencing attitudes to violence against women. *Trauma, Violence and Abuse: A Review Journal, 10*(2), 125–142.

Freedman, J. (2015). *Gendering the international asylums and refugee debate*. Basingstoke, UK: Palgrave Macmillan.

Galtung, J. (1969). Violence, peace, and peace research. *Journal of Peace Research, 6*(3), 167–191.

Garcia-Moreno, C., Jansen, H., Ellsberg, M., Heise, L., & Watts, C. (2006). Prevalence of intimate partner violence: Findings from the WHO multi-country study on women's health and domestic violence. *Lancet, 368*(9543), 1260–1269.
Giddens, A. (1992). *The transformation of intimacy: Sexuality, love and eroticism in modern societies*. Cambridge: Polity.
Gillioz, L., De Puy, J., & Ducret, V. (2000). La violenza domestica in Svizzera: nuovi dati su un fenomeno antico. In P. Romito (Ed.), *Violenze alle donne e risposte delle istituzioni* (pp. 83–96). Milan, Italy: FrancoAngeli.
Giordano, C. (1994). Der Ehrkomplex im Mittelmeerraum: sozialanthropologische Konstruktion oder Grundstruktur mediterraner Lebensform? In L. Vogt & A. Zingerle (Eds.), *Ehre. Archaische Momente in der Moderne*. Frankfurt a.M., Germany: Suhrkamp Verlag.
Gracia, E., & Lila, M. (2015). *Attitudes towards violence against Women in the EU*. European Commission. DG JUST.
Harding, S. G. (1991). *Whose science? Whose knowledge? Thinking from women's lives*. Ithaca, NY: Cornell University Press.
Harding, S. G. (2004). *The feminist standpoint theory reader*. New York/London: Routledge.
Harding, S. G. (2007). Rethinking standpoint epistemology: What is 'strong objectivity'? In K. B. Wray (Ed.), *Knowledge and inquiry: Readings in epistemology* (pp. 352–384). Peterborough, ON: Broadview Press.
Haraway, D. (2004). *The Haraway reader*. New York and London: Routledge.
Kirby, P. (2006). *Vulnerability and violence: The impact of globalization*. London: Pluto Press.
Nixon, J., & Humphreys, C. (2010). Marshalling the evidence: Using intersectionality in the domestic violence frame. *Social Politics, 17*, 137–158.
Nussbaum, M. C. (2000). *Women and human development: The capabilities approach*. New York: University Press.
Peristiany, I. G., & Pitt-Rivers, J. (Eds.). (1991). *Honour and grace in mediterranean society*. Cambridge, UK: Cambridge University Press.
Peristiany, J. G. (Ed.). (1965). *Honor and shame: The values of mediterranean society*. London: Weidenfeld & Nicolson.
Råheim, M., Magnussen, L., Sekse, R., Lunde, A., Jacobsen, T., & Blystad, A. (2016). Researcher–researched relationship in qualitative research: Shifts in positions and researcher vulnerability. *International Journal Qualitative Studies Health Well-being, 11*. Retrieved from https://www.ncbi.nlm.nih.gov/pmc/articles/PMC4910304/
Razack, S. (2011). *La chasse aux musulmans. Evincer les musulmans de l'espace politique*. Montréal, QC: Lux Éditeur.
Sen, A. K. (1999). *Development as freedom*. Oxford, UK: University Press.
Sen, A. K. (2007). *Identity and violence: The illusion of Destiny*. London: Allen Lane.
Walzer, M. (2007). *Thinking politically*. Yale: Yale University Press.
Wolf, W. (1927). *To the lighthouse*. New York: Harcourt, Brace &Co.
Zimmerman, A. M. (2000). Empowerment theory. *Handbook of Psychology Community, 3*, 43–63.

Chapter 5
Violence Through Words: Cultural Aspects and Performative Agency

5.1 A Preamble

Violence has long been considered a *sui generis* topic of the social sciences, almost a corollary of theories dealing with conflict and power (Arendt, 1970; Coser, 1956; Dahrendorf, 1988; Lenski, 1966; Nodstrom, 2004; Wieviorka, 2005). Only recently, some contemporary studies have highlighted, in addition to the procedural transversal nature of the areas invested by it, the unity and constitutive nature of violence which, as a category affects the physical plane of material action, but also the indirect and symbolic area of representation (Bimbi, 2013; Bourdieu, 1998; Collins, 2008; Corradi, 2009).

Violence is simultaneously material and immaterial; therefore, it is expressed both concretely and linguistically. As a constitutive principle of behaviour, unlike aggression (from ad-gradior – "going against" physically and identifiable through concrete actions and reactions), violence highlights a plural phenomenology that permeates actions and intentions, thoughts and linguistic acts, revealing a potent symbolic value at the same time (Bourdieu, 1998).

In the perlocution of linguistic acts, violence is amalgamated with the representations and cultural humus of a society. Besides influencing value constructs and the relational habitus of speakers, when present at an intense level in societies like those of the "Souths", "spoiled by atavistic paradigms of 'honour-and-shame'" (Bartholini, 2015: 12), it helps reinforce cognitive schemata and interpretative models on which individual and collective reasoning is based. Therefore, it impacts on discursive situations and expressive rituals which define "worlds of life" (Habermas, 1981, 1983) which, from the analytical perspective adopted here, mean the Mediterranean. When one thinks of the Mediterranean society one needs to discard any desire for a rational kind of Europeanism and look "in another direction, that of the interminable struggle between conflict and mediation, between the strength of divergent and opposing reasons and the wisdom of measure, between divided truths and opposite

I. Bartholini, *The Trap of Proximity Violence*,
https://doi.org/10.1007/978-3-030-52451-7_5

of the tragedy and the need to mediate encapsulated in the name of this sea, *Mediterranean*" (Cassano, 2007: 79). Violence, therefore, even if "is to be considered a behavioural modality regulated by specific communicative and cultural models" (Bartholini 2013: 204), conveys, in turn, flows of communication as well as the behavioural modalities they help create.

The purpose of the reflections provided below is to detect the double interlink between the symbolic order of violence and the modes of communication adopted in the context of the Mediterranean, by making use of some of the cardinal concepts of contemporary socio-linguistics like agency (Duranti, 2007) and euphemization (Bourdieu, 1993) detectable in certain contemporary written and spoken language procedures amalgamated with some dialectal forms still vivid and in common use locally. This analysis will be carried out through an analysis of some consolidated and ritualized forms of language and daily communication identifiable in the stories of the late, contemporary author, Andrea Camilleri.

5.2 Discourse and the Mediterranean Context

Fairclough (2014) defines discourse as a "special social practice" involving the socially determined use of language. When defining "determined" discourse, he notes how it assumes and reflects an "order of things", a "construction of reality" – as well as a flow of interaction – by means of a range of implications that are not always (or not necessarily) conscious. Although attention to the implications constitutes a heuristic platform for the investigation of fields of discourse analysis, the reflection of the scholar, is, basically, not new. Already Giambattista Vico had advocated the creation of a "mental dictionary" where to safely store "the common meaning of mankind".

It is interesting, however, to point out that those belonging to a specific historical-social context organize their mutual lives according to an order of discourse. This is intended as the set of social practices that interrelate grounded in a specific logic, and referring to social areas (politics, family, the working world), each of which, in turn, contains an order of its own, the outcome of reduced-scale fragmentation of the former which constitutes its matrix. At the same time, the context is constituted by the social situation within which the discourse takes place and provides it with meaningful sense (Fairclough, 1992). In identifying a context, it is necessary to take the spatio-temporal coordinates, institutional conditions, roles, interests involved into account, as well as the different determiners (power relationships, fields of conflict, common sense, hegemonic ideologies, etc.) of a specific locality. In the context of our present reflections, the latter is intended as an incomplete and in-progress realization "involved in the vital processes of the people who compose it" and as an area of the "Mediterranean" characterized by post-modernist thrusts, but also by a contemporary upsurge of the atavistic "honour-and-shame" paradigm (Giordano, 1994; Peristiany, 1965), intended "as its cultural trait, expressed primarily through gender relations oriented towards control over women and the safeguard of the private-public power of men" (Bimbi, 2015: 22). Gender-based violence, in the Mediterranean context of Sicily, combines, therefore, "symbolic aspects with specific socio-cultural matrices, highlighting their contextual interconnections and the categories that support their phenomenal manifestation" (Bartholini 2015: 11), despite the various, differentiated thrusts favoured by the more advanced sectors of this same social milieu.

Discourse as a "social practice" (Fairclough, 2014) performs a crucial function, revealing how violence does not prescind from contexts and situations, from institutional influences, or from the roles and interests in which and through which it is expressed.

Violence, as a modality of relationship, also assumes a function of premise to what people say. This calls into play the distinctions Antonio Gramsci made between "common sense" and "common meaning" (Gramsci, 1952), and how their inversion could subvert the cognitive hierarchies of speakers in a given social system. Words used "for effect", considered "colourful", "insulting", or "hilarious" always contain a certain degree of violence rooted in legacies of common meaning of a Mediterranean type. It is above all a type of gender violence that surfaces in the inter-connection between patriarchalism and neo-patriarchalism of old heritages where the body of women is still considered a *commodity*, an object of "symbolic domination" (Bourdieu, 1998), though not yet of *entitlement*.

Therefore, the performative effects of a violent kind of language and, therefore, of a certain type of communication, impact on both the public and private spheres, on collective representations of the culture, even on the policies and actions of social *governance* in a complex quest for balance between glocal cooperation and competition.

5.3 Agency and the Euphemization Process as Social Practice

It is interesting to point out how contextualized communication determines a procedure for the naturalization of discursive practices which act as a further step in the euphemization process. This common meaning of which individuals are almost always unaware, and which it is extremely difficult to ignore, actually constitutes the structure of daily thinking on the basis of which assessments of *honour-and-shame* are formulated and expressed in daily life. It constitutes a container in which discursive classifications of females are stored.

Common meaning helps, to various extents, to bolster asymmetrical relations, by diverting attention from ideas that might question established power relations and bring to light social and social causes which might destabilize the existing by replacing elements of the paradigm. It is clear, for example, that in an androcentric system every claim to the dignity and acknowledgement of homosexual rights is rejected through processes of euphemization which enhance the role of the traditional family within the educational dynamics of minors. *Euphemization* is a socio-linguistic process but also the result of a compromise between what is known as an *expressive interest* (the need to communicate what needs to be communicated) and censorship within the field where linguistic expression takes shape.

Euphemized speech, according to Bourdieu, exerts symbolic violence upon agents when a statement "declares that it is not what it really is" (Bourdieu, 1993: 90–93). Following this line of thought, one could assume that language acts as a mirror image of the world of life and that the processes of language used reflect the behavioural and cognitive mechanisms of those who use the language (Searle, 1972) in that specific *localité*. It is not actually an exact image; it refers, rather, to future constructs and is rooted in historically hypostatized connections.

The ways in which particular meanings are associated with particular phenomena can provide insight into the culture of the speakers of a given variety of language. There are also some ideological peculiarities that are evident in the co-occurrence of particular linguistic expressions. It may be assumed, therefore, that sets of words which usually co-occur in given contexts should carry a fair amount of contextual implications. This is so. The European Mediterranean is still a place where relational modes, attitudes, and communication codes referring to the symbolic male universe still prevail, creating an organizational context hostile to women. In this sense, the words are contextual and projective because the discourse deriving from them provides a thematization, that is, the establishment not only of the object but also of the framework which outlines the reality in a certain way by selecting aspects considered appropriate to highlight.

Precisely because language is social action, studies regarding the use of language explain how violence emerges in dialogical form starting with the daily linguistic interactions inherent within a context. The lexicon comprising commonly used vocabulary also establishes ways of acting and interacting with others and with things.

From this point of view, the everyday spoken form of the Sicilian dialect contains some "ergative marks" (Duranti, 1994), meaning grammatical forms present in some languages used to treat the subjects of transitive verbs differently from the subjects of intransitive verbs. Duranti, studying the Samoan community, explains how the most powerful among these people are more likely use an ergative mark whenever they wish to accuse someone of having intentionally committed some iniquity, considering it better suited to denote the agency producing certain effects in terms of responsibility and the sanctionability of the action. However, they may also mitigate and, therefore, euphemize the action to which they refer.

What determines agency, "the power of words", or the performative effectiveness of an illocutionary act does not lie so much in the words themselves, but in some conditions that may be summed up as an authority. The "power of words", or the success of the statements Bourdieu calls "actions of social magic", does not depend on whether they are understood, but, rather, on the authoritativeness and/or (violent) authority of those authorized or acknowledged, therefore, permitted to utter such "perlocutive communicative acts". The latter are concentrations of symbolic capital accumulated in the fissures of those "vital worlds" which, in our case, comprise Mediterranean identity.

Very recently, S. Gesuato (2003a, 2003b) observed that although the terms men, women, boy, and girl can be used within the same areas of speech and associated with similar topics and concepts, the frequency of their occurrence within these domains may prove very different. Males were often described with reference to notions of power while feminine language modifiers emphasize the referent's beauty, age, and physical attributes, while most male modifiers indicate the general notion of male attractiveness. In addition, the wife/wives lexeme is often modified by attributes emphasizing traditional female roles. As we shall see later, in euphemized and Mediterranean contexts of discursive domains (therefore, where the neo-patriarchal paradigm of honour-and-shame applies), the verbal forms referred to a husband convey notions of activity, positivity, and cognitive ability, while the co-occurring lexical items referred to a wife indicate notions of passivity, negativity, and physicality by "gender-neutral" shifting of the latter's habitus to attitudes that either echo that of males by making differences imperceptible or assuming a naturalized attitude implying the free circulation of female erotic capital.

In the following pages, I shall endeavour to highlight how language, while aspiring to gender neutrality, actually stigmatizes elements of gender discontinuity by imposing sexist logic. It does so precisely by using recurrent ergative marks comprising the spoken language which were transferred into the written language made universally interpretable thanks to the stories of Andrea Camilleri and in the wake of a Mediterranean tradition consolidated by Verga, Bufalino, Sciascia, and numerous other writers. From this point of view, writing not only preserves the knowledge "of southern thinking (which) explicitly claims the existence of a connection between the Italian south and the south of the world" (Cassano, 1996: IX), but is also capable of bestowing credit on lexemes and periphrases. This vital form of appropriation is a trait of this kind of operation, since by drawing from texts, one acquires knowledge, a view of the whole world, potentially providing the opportunity to generate further discourse and shape other ways of acting and living. Lexical transformations show that the history of the meanings to which words refer and of the concepts they conserve, do not aim at their euphemization, nor do they denote increasing rationality (Foucault, 1971). According to Fairclough (1991), the process of appropriation operates in the dual colonization/emancipation sense, but, more often than not, it ends up by "conditioning" those who use it within a given context. In reality, on the basis of the logic of domination, language imposes an ideology that foresees both the agency of the dominators and the euphemization of the dominated as well as of the spectators within the dynamics of a symbolic domination of an androcentric kind. The internalization of feelings of self-evaluation and self-denigration is often perpetuated spontaneously by those very women who use the dominant categories applying them to women themselves. On the other hand, "symbolic domination cannot be exercised without the contribution of those submitted to it" (Bourdieu, 1998: 3).

5.4 Camilleri's Vocabulary: A Late Modern Mirror of the Mediterranean Representation of Women

Camilleri's merit lies in his prose which avails itself of a Sicilian dialect intimately integrated with standard Italian and used to convey both the account provided by the narrating voice and the dialogues. He used a Sicilian lexicon leaving the syntax unchanged, which is why dialectal terms are widespread throughout his novels while the grammar remains that of the official language. The textual consistency of Camilleri's stories lies in their representations of experiences and activities, on the one hand, and in the construction of roles and social relations on the other. In his delivery of dialectal words with high symbolic violence content, we found it interesting to peruse and subdivide, by gender, some of the terms used most frequently by the author. Those reported in this first perusal are taken from the novel entitled *La forma dell'acqua* [The shape of water], published in 1994, the first of the fortunate series featuring Police-Commissioner Montalbano.

It is interesting to observe the variety with which women are indicated in the dialect used in Camillieri's works. On the one hand, this testifies to the linguistic richness of the Sicilian language, though, on the other – in a selection of the emblematic material which best underlines the characterizing elements of the agency and euphemization process – they highlight a stratification referring not only to social determinants but also to specifics of sexuality linked to the "honour-and-shame" cultural paradigm.

Picciotta (young one/lass/lassie): "*Prima dell'ingegnere ho quella picciotta di una ventina d'anni (...)*" (Camilleri 1995: 25)

[Before the engineer I have that twenty-year-old-ish *young lass*]

Signora (lady; married woman; madam/ma'am); signuri (Mr and Mrs, meaning "respectable" people/gentlefolk): *"Mi perdoni, signora, cercavo i signori Montaperto"*. [Excuse me ma'am, I was looking for Mr and Mrs Montaperto]

"Signuri Montaperto? Ca quali signuri! Chiddri munnizzari vastasi sunnu!" (Ibidem: 148).

[*Mr and Mrs* Montaperto? What *Mr and Mrs*! *Vulgar rubbish collectors that's all they are*!]

Moglie (wife): *"Lunidia a matinu prestu, alla mànnara (...) Nonsi, sulu a me muglieri."* (Ibidem: 64)

[Monday morning early, at the sheepfold (...) No sir, only to my wife]

Femmina (female); *Fimmina* (piece of skirt/ broad/bird):

"*Quando hanno finito, la femmina ha aperto lo sportello e è scesa, si è aggiustata la gonna, ha richiuso. L'uomo, invece di rimettere in moto e partire, se n'è rimasto al suo posto, la testa appoggiata all'indietro* (ibidem: 48).

[When they finished, the female opened the door and got out, fixed her skirt, closed [the door] again. Instead of restarting and leaving, the man remained with his head leaning backwards.

> *La femmina è passata rasente la macchina di Carmen e proprio in quel momento è stata pigliata in pieno dai fari di un'automobile. Era una bella fimmina, bionda, elegante*" (ibidem: 49).
>
> The female passed close to Carmen's car and just them she was lit up fully by the headlights of a car. She was a beautiful *piece of skirt*, blonde, elegant]

Camilleri's women can be located within a sexist universe thematized by three general isotopies: the amorous, the sexual, the culinary, which hardly ever overlap but which constitute the frame of the text, therefore, of the author's discourse.

They are "wives/mothers" (Livia and the housekeeper, Adelina) or women to be courted, like in *Il ladro di merendine* [The Snack Thief] the young Mrs Gulisano, whores (Karima) or undesirable women (the "Piccirillos" and Mrs. Pinna with her "tree trunk legs").

Only older women seem to now deserve at times detached respect (like Aisha or the school-marm Vasile Cozzo), at others with asexual contempt (Mrs. Lapecora).

Even the dialectal language which often accompanies the women described in Camilleri's stories connotes a violent value which describes a cultural setting of backwardness and sexism. Woman is a "topic", an ideal-typical model, with which to stigmatize the feminine universe. On the contrary, the men are almost always "public figures", in other words, professionals: policemen, professors, security guards ... mafia and criminals who impose and "authoritatively" denote a certain view of the social world. They exercise the power of "ergative marks", especially when dealing with women, sometimes with homosexuals, in the frequently unmindful agency of euphemization.

Trying to highlight the emblematic material that best foregrounds elements which characterize Mediterranean discourse and the links in the "dialect-sexism-symbolic-violence" chain, we wish to present in the table below, some of the lexemes frequently used in Camillieri's corpus:

Table 5.1 provides some examples of nouns (masculine and feminine) associated with the corresponding verb whose meanings, often allegorical, at times figured, and contain, in our opinion a high degree of symbolic violence both on the level of agency and on the place of ergative marks.

For example, with regard to the verb "amminchiare", it is Camilleri himself, in *Il gioco della mosca* [The game of the fly] who provides the following definition: "It is said that a man is 'amminchiato' when he stubbornly insists on a point that is difficult to sustain in the light of reason".

Again, in the collection of anecdotes, regarding the verb "annacare", the writer describes the different *gender-oriented* interpretations of the term: "It is universal belief that a woman who 'annacas' everyone while walking, publicly proclaims her lack of seriousness". When applied to a man the issue becomes more complex. "I asked the mayor for a favour and he nodded at me for a year without concluding: he deluded me, cradled my hope and ultimately made fun of me".

The verb "murritiare" takes on different meanings depending on the subject: in the case of a woman it means "to tease, provoke" and is charged with clear sexual references. In the case of a man, it implies "seeking, trying, searching with curiosity and tenacity" (Table 5.2).

Table 5.1 Esempi di lessemi dialettali gender oriented

Substantive	Verb	Grammatical value/ semantic value
Spinno: desire or nostalgia	*Spinnare*: strongly desire	Masculine/ Masculine
Pirtusa: holes	*Spirtusare*: create a hole	Masculine/ Masculine
Spercio: desire	*Sperciare*: want, desire, feel like	Masculine/ Masculine
Fissa: foolish, stupid, or female sexual organ	*Fissiarsela*: linger, waste time	Feminine/ Masculine
Annacata: swinging; rocking (e.g. a cradle); swaying (hips; buttocks)	*Annacare*: cradle, waste time, fiddle, sway, deceive	Feminine/ Masculine-Feminine
Garruso: passive homosexual	*Garrusiare:* behave astutely and ambiguously	Masculine/ Masculine
*Minchia**: inactive male organ	*Amminchiare*: be discouraged, regret temporarily, not grasp a simple concept	Feminine/ Masculine
Murritiuso: one who never stands still or touches everything; even "those suffering from haemorrhoids"	*Murritiare*: annoy, but also joke using one's hands or words; "provoke"	Feminine/ Masculine-Feminine

Table 5.2 Examples of gender-oriented lemmatic dialectal variations

Feminine noun or adjective	Masculine noun or adjective	Semantic predominance
Passuluna dried black olives.	*Passulune*: of a passive or dull man or boy	Injurious distortion of the feminine noun *uva passula* meaning raisin
*Minchia**: masculine male organ	*Minchione*: of a man or boy, passive or dull	Injurious distortion of the masculine noun declined in the feminine gender
Caiorda: prostitute, dirty, sordid, "slut"	*Caiordo*: dirty, sordid	Injurious distortion of the feminine substantivated adjective

From the analysis of these two tables – where for the sake of methodological convenience we have placed some of the terms used in the contemporary language spoken in Palermo – the dynamics of symbolic violence contained in the words and sexual references listed is immediate. Beyond these examples, Camilleri's Sicilian-Italian vocabulary conveys details of an infinity of expressions linked with a patriarchal culture based on a legacy of "shame-and-honour". From this wholly Mediterranean perspective, the discourse includes not only representations of what people are like or of the construction of people and events, but also of the imaginary, that is, views of how what is described and narrated might or should be.

It is also interesting to highlight, from our point of view, how the linguistic/cultural links between the Sicilian dialect and the Italian language are acknowledged by the Legislator. In 1981, the Sicilian Parliament approved a regional law, n° 85, which provided that it "intended to encourage the study of the Sicilian dialect and the languages of the ethnic minorities in the island's schools". The text of the law was inspired by the dictates of the Decrees issued in 1974 (art. 12 paragraph 3 of the DM n. 416/1974) where "the inclusion, in school programmes, of studies and research useful to a better knowledge of local realities" was recommended having been inspired by bill n° 731 of a few years earlier, presented by Pier Santi Mattarella. In its premise, the law stated that "The dialect needs to be intended in purely cultural terms, given that for every people it represents the source of its culture, the possibility of being recognized within its own ethnic group due to the tongue in which it expresses itself, the need to safeguard its own traditions of customs, habits and language, the need to present itself in the present by means of its past and find its own identity". From this point of view, Camilleri's prose enlivens the "hidden" power of linguistic traditions, because although the implications relating to power relations are not explicit, they nevertheless become "universal common meaning". Cultural consent, discursive centrality, institutionalization, and the marginalization or delegitimization of alternatives are widely documented features of socially dominant masculinities (Connell & Messerschmidt, 2005).

5.5 Conclusions

Violence, as a unitary (Corradi, 2009) and constitutive (Bartholini, 2013) phenomenon, if on the one hand, it underpins some types of deviant relationships which rest upon it, on the other, it preserves and confirms some expressions that due to the high degree of agency of which they are woven, define the performative impact of communication. Violent words produce structural and long-term consequences because they act through knowledge and beliefs, impacting on interpersonal relationships and the social development of institutions and society which confirm that between men and women there has been a long, indisputable asymmetry of power, status, resources, supported by attitudes and behaviour which, from time to time, has been defined as male chauvinism, sexism, and machoism.

Language has born witness to the fact that it has been "located" in the Mediterranean and that it may also be "ritualized" at the communicative level and "procrastinated ad interim" through the use of ergative marking.

From a socio-linguistic point of view, while the situation is the unit of analysis of non-random action, when communicative acts use lexemes with high degrees of symbolic significance, they become veritable gender-oriented rituals. In communication, some lexemes with a strong symbolic-emotional value – therefore performative – define the transition from situation to ritual. When this transition occurs, it is precisely because of these "strong" words which retain a certain degree of "meaningfulness and/or violence" within them. The latter combines symbolic aspects with specific socio-cultural matrices, highlighting the interconnections between signifiers and significances, and permits their attribution to those who exercise or undergo specific aspects of identity (Bartholini, 2015).

Analysing some lexemes, by means of a heuristic procedure capable of revealing degrees of symbolic violence contained in the discursive practices related to their use, has allowed us to highlight some of the links underlying inter-gender and inter-generational relationships within a specific situational and/or ritual cross-section of Mediterranean Sicily by emphasizing the links it still holds with the *honour-and-shame* paradigm which thrived in a place of "land and sea. With a hinterland vast enough to allow the germs of a peasant culture to intertwine and interweave with those of a more miscellaneous and dynamic culture typical of fishermen and sailors" (Camilleri, 1995: 11).

References

Arendt, H. (1970). *On violence*. New York: Harvest/Harcourt Brace & Company.
Bartholini, I. (Ed.). (2015). *Violenza di genere e percorsi mediterranei. Voci, saperi, uscite*. Milan, Italy: Guerini e Associati.
Bartholini, I. (2013). *Violenza di prossimità. La vittima, il carnefice e il "grande occhio"*. Milan, Italy: FrancoAngeli.
Bimbi, F. (Ed.). (2013). *Agency of migrant Women against gender violence. Final comparative report of the project* "speak out! Empowering migrant, refugee and ethnic minority women against gender violence in Europe", co-founded by EU for the Daphne Programme, AB Edizioni-Alphabeta Verlag, Bolzano.
Bimbi, F. (2015). Onore-e-vergogna. Il ritorno di un paradigma mediterraneo nel dibattito europeo. In I. Bartholini (Ed.), *Violenza di genere e percorsi mediterranei. Voci, saper, uscite* (pp. 27–44). Milan, Italy: Guerini e Associati.
Bourdieu, P. (1993). *La Misère du monde*. Paris: Editions de Seuil.
Bourdieu, P. (1998). *Masculine domination*. Stanford, CA: Stanford University Press.
Camilleri, A. (1995). *Il gioco della mosca*. Palermo, Italy: Sellerio.
Cassano, F. (1996). *Il pensiero meridiano*. Rome, Italy/Bari, Italy: Laterza.
Cassano, F. (2007). Necessità del Mediterraneo. In F. Cassano e D. Zolo (a cura di), *L'alternativa mediterranea* (pp. 8–110). Milan, Italy: Feltrinelli.
Collins, R. (2008). *Violence. A micro-sociological theory*. Princeton, NJ: University Press.
Connell, R. W., & Messerschmidt, J. W. (2005). Hegemonic masculinity: Rethinking the concept. *Gender and Society, 1*, 829–859.
Corradi, C. (2009). *Sociologia della violenza. Modernità, identità, potere*. Rome, Italy: Meltemi.
Coser, L. A. (1956). *The functions of social conflicts*. Glencoe, Scotland: The Free Press.
Dahrendorf, R. (1988). *The modern social conflict*. New York: Weidenfield & Nicholson (trad. it.: *Il conflitto sociale nella modernità*, Laterza, Rome-Bari, 1989).
Duranti, A. (1994). *From grammar to politics: Linguistic anthropology in a Western Samoan Village*. Berkeley, CA: University of California Press.
Duranti, A. (2007). *Etnopragmatica. La forza nel parlare*. Rome, Italy: Carocci Editore.
Fairclough, N. (1991). *Discourse and social change*. Cambridge, UK: Polity Press.
Fairclough, N. (1992). *Critical language awareness*. Harlow, UK/London: Longman.
Fairclough, N. (2014). *Language and power*. Harlow, UK/London: Longman (3rd edition, 1989 1st edition).
Foucault, M. (1971). *L'ordre du discours*. Paris, France: Gallimard, Paris.
Gesuato, S. (2003a). The company women and men keep: What collocations can reveal about culture. In D. Archer, P. Rayson, A. Wilson, & T. McEnery (Eds.), *Proceedings of the Corpus linguistics conference* (pp. 253–262). Lancaster, PA: Lancaster University.

Gesuato, S. (2003b). The company women and men keep: What collocations can reveal about culture. In D. Archer, P. Rayson, A. Wilson, & T. McEnery (Eds.), *Proceedings of the Corpus linguistics conference* (pp. 253–271). Lancaster, PA: Lancaster University.

Giordano, C. (1994). Der Ehrkomplex im Mittelmeerraum: sozialanthropologische Konstruktion oder Grundstruktur mediterraner Lebensform? In L. Vogt & A. Zingerle (Eds.), *Ehre. Archaische Momente in der Moderne* (pp. 172–192). Frankfurt a.M., Germany: Suhrkamp Verlag.

Gramsci, A. (1952). *Il materialismo storico e la filosofia di Benedetto Croce*. Turin, Italy: Einaudi.

Habermas, J. (1981). *Theorie des kommunikativen Handelns*: Bd. I. *Handlungsratio nalität und gesellschaftliche Rationalisierung*: Bd. II. *Zur Kritik der funktionalistischen Vernunft*. Frankfurt a.M., Germany: Suhrkamp Verlag.

Habermas, J. (1983). *Moralbewusstsein und kommunikatives Handeln*. Frankfurt a.M., Germany: Suhrkamp Verlag.

Lenski, G. E. (1966). *Power and privilege: A theory of social stratification*. New York: McGraw-Hill Book Company.

Nodstrom, C. (2004). *Shadows of war: Violence, power and international profiteering in the twenty-first century*. Berkeley, CA: University of California Press.

Peristiany, J. G. (Ed.). (1965). *Honor and shame: The values of Mediterranean society*. London: Weidenfeld & Nicolson.

Searle, J. (1972). *Speech acts: An essay on the philosophy of language*. Cambridge, UK: Cambridge University Press.

Wieviorka, M. (2005). *La Violence*. Paris, France: Hachette.

Chapter 6
European Mediterranean Women and the "Showdown" Between Public Emancipation and Private Self-oppression

6.1 Public Discourse and Mediterraneanness in Europe

Today, there is no such thing as a single culturally dominant West but many Wests and "Western souths". There is an Atlantic Europe and a Mediterranean Europe, the latter bordering on the world of Islam, in its Arabic, Persian, Kurdish, and Turkish variants (Cassano & Zolo, 2007). Proximity violence may be defined primarily as a cultural problem, structured around ways of constructing the role of women and gender relationships within a given social context (Monckton-Smith, 2012).

The pathways of a "dominant" and an "underground" culture intersect. The former is of a late-modern type, widely acknowledged; the other, equally present and bearing with it, neo-patriarchal implications. The former officially rejects gender-based violence in all its forms; the other rejects it but, at the same time, justifies it. On the one hand, we endorsed paradigm of the free circulation of female erotic capital; on the other, the reaffirmation of oppressive family ties (Bimbi, 2015). Their frames of presentation and legitimization concern the same sphere of culturally extended influence existing between Europe and the Mediterranean countries. Their interactive game of mirrors, Atlantic culture postmodern (Sassen, 1999) – and Mediterranean culture – still strongly influenced by premodern drifts (Giordano, 2005) – have produced broad gaps of discontinuity between public discourse and discourse related to private or community customs. In the Mediterranean area the "honour-shame" paradigm (Bimbi, 2015; Giordano, 2005; Peristiany, 1965), aimed at the control of women who "belong" to a man as partner, bride, fiancée, and even as ex-partner, is still a prevalent feature of individual research projects, supported by the long sequence of femicides which occur daily in the area. *Honour-related* crimes as an extreme form of gender-based violence following a woman's separation from or abandonment of a man inform the idea that recognition of the male continues to pass through affirmation of his dominion over women.

I. Bartholini, *The Trap of Proximity Violence*,
https://doi.org/10.1007/978-3-030-52451-7_6

The hierarchy of masculinities is a pattern of hegemony, not a pattern of simple nomination based on force. Cultural consent, discursive centrality, institutionalization, and the marginalization or delegitimation of alternatives are widely documented features of socially dominant masculinities (Connell & Messerschmidt, 2005).

Despite female emancipation, the body of a woman continues to be an instrument used to assert male dominion which, the more it is scaled down in the public sphere, the more it assumes attitudes of vehemence within the intimate and private spheres. "This body of work erected a sharp divide between the culture of northern and southern Europe by separating 'moderns' from those were deemed 'non-yet-moderns'" (Greverus, Romhild, & Welz, 2001: 3). This process outsources personal identity, meaning that one sees oneself primarily through the eyes of the other (Bartholini, 2013) while also being acknowledged by the other (Honneth, 1995). The process of the outsourcing of personal identity is not new to sociological analysis and can be used to throw light on the relationship between gender violence and the exteriority/fragility of self-representations in the world of "Mediterranean" men who commit feminicides and perpetrate family violence.

From this angle, proximity violence may be defined as the effect of a dyscrasia between cultural models that have not been sufficiently harmonized and which act as a barrier to the model of "converging love, (which) is in a certain sense the opposite of projective identification" (Giddens, 1992: 72). Proximity violence has become an "in-between phenomenon", the understanding of which permits us to intercept the inconsistencies arising between female emancipation at the public level and the cultural legacies of the Mediterranean. These legacies are fostered also by the presence of retrograde migrant cultures which are also capable of exercising indirect influence over indigenous cultural representations. The latter, while siding with modernity, find it difficult to abandon the legacies of the past, and end up by fomenting conflict between the various strands of public discourse.

The intersection between discontinuous cultural paradigms on the diachronic plane and parallel ones on the synchronic plane highlights the need to:

(a) Tackle, by means of reflective openness, divergent cultural paradigms, but also attempts made on several fronts to bring the hands of the historical-social clock back to an archaic and premodern dimension of community life.
(b) Perceive the repeated attempts made to reject pluralistic and post-materialistic values by imposing – even in a skulking manner – neo-patriarchal values boosted by drifts of a Mediterranean culture that become radical and fundamentalist in their opposition to processes of Western modernization.

Mediterranean culture even if in the minority assumes more aggressive positions and, therefore, is capable of suggesting and creating in the intimate sphere conditions incongruent with the conquests females have made in the public sphere. All this in favour of a subjective well-being of a male variety, though obtained in captivity, brings men in the spotlight of that infinitely small audience – small but absolutely necessary – where the Other than self, in the role of the closest to him – the partner – is essential.

In this chapter, we shall try to untie some of the knots of the relationship existing between proximity violence, "adaptive preferences", and "corrosive disadvantages" within the private sphere, which are totally at odds with social conquest and are, on the contrary, the outcome of "social constructs" (Berger & Luckmann, 2000) haphazardly internalized and rooted in their universe of meaning.

6.2 A Late Unfinished Modernity Amid Postmodernist Thrusts and Mediterranean Heritage

In the contemporary West, some of the objectives prompting transition towards a political, economic, and cultural post-modernization of society seem to have been achieved (Balandier, 1994; Bauman, 2000; Beck, 1998; Giddens, 1992; Inglehart, 2018); among these, the emancipation of women and their inclusion in full in the public sphere of the professions. The so-called phenomenon of "feminization of the workforce" dates back to the 1950s, but it is only in recent years that gender segregation has given way to effective participation by women at all levels. Their visibility on the labour market represents a significant degree of discontinuity due to the effects produced not only with respect to the past, but in the corporate balances and *governance* structures that have arisen (Reyneri, 2011; Saraceno & Keck 2011). The entry of women into the world of the liberal professions, into employment, trade, and the services has also required a review of welfare policies and conciliation plans regarding the family system. It has also led to a deeper analysis of the balances upon which the dynamics of gender relations and identities are based, precisely by virtue of the redefinition of the no-longer hegemonic, exclusive functions of men in public life, and the renegotiation of the respective roles of a couple within a relationship.

If, on the one hand, female emancipation has constituted an authentic revolution – as well as an element of breach with the past – within the family context, we find, on the contrary, strong regressive tensions, aimed at re-establishing a "restorative balance" which in the intimate sphere, restores to the male partner those signs of power which have disappeared along with the loss of his role as *male breadwinner* (Bartholini, 2014). These attempts, supported by traditional practices and codes of inspired by religion, find their extreme expression in proximity violence. It deconstructs the dynamics upon which relationships of intimacy are based, which, by definition "is above all a question of emotional communication with oneself and with others in a context of equality" (Giddens, 2000: 142) by imposing asymmetry and subordination. Although *gender violence* (or proximity violence as it would be more appropriate to call it) has been considered so far an integral part of definitions of conflict and power, it is, nonetheless, from a culturalist perspective, a category capable of explaining interpersonal dynamics at both micro (Collins, 2008; Wright & Decker, 1997) and macro-sociological level (Balibar, 2001; Thapar-Björkert, 2007), precisely because in it old legacies and new forms of female and male capacity converge to hinder the possibility of establishing "converging relationships" (Giddens, 2000).

The reappearance and, under certain conditions, the imposition of neo-patriarchal and neo-macho revanches within intimate relationships (Bartholini, 2015, 2019; Walter, 2010) leads us to see how, in actual fact, "we have not gone beyond modernity; on the contrary, we are in the midst of a phase of radicalisation of modernity" (Giddens, 2000: 57), and note that Modernity is still an "unfinished project" (Habermas, 1985) where emancipation has not taken place *wholly*, but in discontinuous watertight compartments. Although our nation is founded on the equality of all citizens, gender equality frequently turns the division of tasks within a couple's relationship into an increase in the number of tasks assigned to women as a result of her equal rights and duties which, in reality, spell double work for her both at home and in the workplace, poorly backed by still inadequate practices of conciliation.

In addition, her emancipation and the flexibility of her work in the public sphere finds its counterpart in the *disembedding* of her interpersonal relationships. If women and men are engaged, on the one hand, in catering for the challenges of an increasingly flexible and *whippy* labour market on the other, they are exposed to a similar kind of elasticity in their intimate relationships which clashes, however, with other representations of the stability and continuity that relationships involving couples present in their imaginations. If the procedural elements of public life may be contained by rationality, the emotional inclinations on which personal balance is based are far less manageable. This dyscrasia causes tensions that are sometimes irreducible within the relationships of couples where legacies and representations of the past are still vivid (Hanmer & Itzin, 2001) and capable of generating violence in an attempt to keep the relationship standing. It is for this precise reason that proximity violence and emotional oppression (itself the product of relational oppression) act as authentic strategies for the maintenance of relationships that weaken and/or overwhelm the capacity for autonomy and dignity widely applied by women in the public sphere.

The full participation of women in the world of work seems not to correspond, therefore, to acknowledgement of their role and dignity within the intimate sphere, but rather to greater exploitation of their emotional-affective resources by employment of a code of symbolic representation that amalgamates the lexicon of femininity with a more covert misogynous and neo-patriarchal one, however disguised and "gilded" by values like fidelity, reciprocity, and free donation. All this – and this is our thesis – has generated veritable "corrosive disadvantages" to the detriment of all those women hovering in the balance, in their "amphibiotic habitus" on the brink between emancipation and emotional subordination to traditional representations.

6.3 Public Emancipation and Private Oppression

If women, despite the difficulties that the various sectors underline, are actively engaged in their working lives to confirm roles and functions, skills and competences denied them in the past or undervalued by a hegemonic male society; in their private life they are often held hostage by emotions associated with archaic representations of their roles as women and partners, mothers and lovers, which turn into "corrosive disadvantages" (Nussbaum, 2016). While the working world assumes *gender neutrality* as a relational model and skill as the main key to acquisition of position within the labour market, the private sphere is exposed to influences of a different nature, which may be defined in the reference area of the gender violence and emotional dynamics which Collins (2008) called "forward panic", Nussbaum *hot emotion* (2004) which, at the same time was *rhythmic and strongly entraining emotion* (Collins, 2008). The possible re-establishment of mechanisms of domination by action at psychological level takes place by bringing into play emotional energies that underlie the interpersonal dimension of Eros and affectivity, which influence the subjectivity of the victims and their mental makeup, when categorizing, perceiving, and assessing (Gracia & Lila, 2015).

The dynamic between dyads we consider oppositional, broadly speaking – public sphere–private sphere, autonomy-dependence, symmetry-subalternity, subjectivity-social organization – suggests that "we are entering an era where the consequences of modernity are (actually) made increasingly radical" (Giddens, 1992: 57); radical, therefore, double, albeit ambiguous, as dangers and risks increase precisely within that part of society which seemed to have redeemed itself from a pre-modern destiny, according to which gender was the fundamental principle of the regulation of social life, behaviour and power relationships, to the detriment of women who show acceptance and tolerance attitudes still quite widespread.

Violence within couple relationships releases a paradoxically coagulating and stabilizing kind of action, liturgically ritualized over time and ranging from preparation (threats, silences, blackmail, dis-confirmation. and disappointed responses) to the explosion of violence itself. If *gender violence*, in its pre-modern perspective stemmed from the fundamental and universal inequality existing between men and women, and from the subordination of the latter to the former (Bimbi, 2003), in its contemporary form, it surfaces explicitly, above all, as repeated attempts to regain positions of dominion men have lost and as the emotional blackmail to which women condemn themselves due to premodern (Kimmel, 2000) and modern (Pinker, 2011) cultural representations still present in Mediterranean culture. If proximity violence, in its classical conception, was used as a tool aimed at subordinating women to the will of males, today it has a social force charged with meaning (Corradi, 2009), endowed with the ability to structure reality by rebalancing in private the loss of status and identity men have experienced in the public sphere as a result of female emancipation (Bartholini, 2015).

Proximity violence therefore:

1. is partly the product of the merging of incompatible cultural paradigms within the same territorial area;
2. is, in part, the product of attempts made to reaffirm that "male domination" (Bourdieu, 1998) undermined by the professional emancipation of women paralleled by their personal independence;

3. is a constitutive – therefore, institutional – aspect of a relationship and, as such, increasingly involves the partner or former partner and almost never a woman who is an outsider, therefore external to the sphere of relational acknowledgement.

A few years ago, Giddens wrote that "today's separating and divorcing society has become the consequence rather than the cause of the birth of converging love [...]. Converging love is active, contingent love and does not rhyme, therefore, with 'forever' and 'one and only'" (Giddens, 1992: 72). Today, we are witnessing the emergence of asymmetrical and oppressive relationships, where the unequal divergence between roles is the product of a type of oppression that Mediterranean-Western women help create for themselves.

6.4 Women's Amphibiotic Habitat

It is not simply an attempt to impose outdated models, but rather the configuration of attitudes and behaviour that tend towards the "spontaneous" acceptance of dynamics of subordination by women and of psychological domination as the only tool used by men against their partner to recover their former status. This creates veritable communicative aphasia within the couple where the woman is silent, obfuscates her needs, limits her expectations, though fully aware of her ability to assert her reasons and needs. So, it is not a question of not "feeling able", but of women voluntarily accepting an underlying subordinate habitus in their private lives, which facilitates the exercise of violence by men. In these cases, the goal is to have the partners converge on common denominator which maintains the relationship and keeps it in time (Bartholini, 2015). If we add the increasingly mythical aspiration by women to "completeness of identity" by means of a personal type of realization combining professional skills in the workplace and personal skills within the private marital sphere, which becomes a *conditio* sine qua non of effective social recognition of women. The common opinion today is that a woman who renounces or places a stable partnership in the background is socially only a woman by halves. Economic and professional autonomy becomes a sword of Damocles forcing women to demonstrate their ability to combine the skills of partner and mother with those of *female breadwinner*. The desire to comply with the emancipatory offices of the public and those of the traditional-conservative private spheres is transformed into a state of veritable emotional self-impoundment which obliges women to tumble cruelly; the more they waver on the wire like the tight-rope-walkers in a Chagall painting, the more likely they are to fall.

Furthermore, changes in mass values and their progressive liquefaction go hand in hand with attempts made to hybridize value and belief systems – those of the Mediterranean and of the Atlantic – due to migration. This favours a reshuffling of inter-gender habituses and attitudes which often translate into the adoption of behaviour and attitudes aimed at facilitating the compliance of women and, in some cases, acceptance of their partners' attempts to reaffirm their *male domination* within the relationship. The product of this voluntary attuning to self-subordination to male *revanches* provides women with that emotional gratification which derives from feeling having been capable of maintaining the relationship even at the cost of "places between parentheses" those very abilities asserted in the public sphere (Bartholini, 2016).

As far as women are concerned, it is a question of a truly **amphibiotic habitus** (from *amphibolía*, "uncertainty", and *lógos*, "discourse"), double in nature and uncertain in its narration. According to Bourdieu habitus, as a "structured structure" "has a bond of dependence with the social world" (Bourdieu, 1979: 191) which cannot be modified and, as a "structuring structure", "organises practices and perceptions of practices" (ibidem). At the same time, however, it refers to "a system of patterns of perception, thought and action acquired permanently and generated by objective conditions, which tend to persist even after these conditions have changed" (ibidem). In this sense, the female habitus, precisely because it is determined, in part, by social structures and, in part, by conflicting representations, creates communicational dystonies that re-accommodate themselves only in acceptance of the incongruent behaviour that follows and limits the primary ability to feel. The transition from the paradigm of addiction, typical of patriarchal cultures, to the paradigm of emancipation, brings in its wake the detritus of an unfinished revolution which transforms the goals achieved by women in the public sphere into a more pernicious identity unease in the private sphere compared to disappointed expectations regarding a female role congruent with the patriarchal representations still present in late-modern men and women.

What, in the public sector constitutes an indisputable reality within, that is, acquired equality of tasks and functions between genders, in the private sphere, eclipses the persistence of that asymmetry of roles justified by archaic cultural representations, often handed down unconsciously and which impacts upon the emotional sphere of women. It is often a sort of emotional self-requisition – which limits their ability to feel and will something women practice for themselves and by themselves – where internalizations of premodern representations of "how" a woman should be destined mother and companion prevail, however. In other extreme forms, these same women subject themselves to a sort of "modern sacrifice" involving intimate violence where neo-patriarchal reverberations of *male domination*, practices of empathic-oppressive delegitimization of ability and identity converge.

6.5 Corrosive Capacities and Disadvantages

According to a recent *Declaration on Femicide in the United Nations Commission on Crime Prevention and Criminal Justice* (2013) "the form of the murder of a female as a result of domestic violence by an intimate partner (husbands and lovers, ex-husbands and ex-lovers)", also because of that symbolic violence widespread in daily representations which frequently prevents women from considering themselves bearers of rights and people of equal dignity and value.

In this sense, it is opportune to emphasize once again how *gender violence* is proximity violence. The possibility of its implementation is subject to the identity of the perpetrator who is hardly ever a stranger to the victim. However, if he is a *proximus*, companion, boyfriend or husband, the possibility of a hidden reason, therefore, a possible narration of the facts extraneous to pure and simple victim–perpetrator dichotomy, winds its way into public perception, transforming the victim into a quasi-victim and the perpetrator in a subject put to the test by the conflicting and contradictory effects of the partner's double habitus. Furthermore, while indicating a non-random assault, which is actually repeated and continued at various levels, the violence is legitimized within an oppressive context determined by the degree of intimacy of the proximate subjects co-participating as partners in the relationship.

What justifies *gender violence* is its proximal character, a term that derives from *proximus* and refers to that absolute superlative indicating the person closest to another. This explains the type of relationship in which subjects are mutually linked by a closeness deriving from "sharing an emotional experience" (Collins, 2008). The proximus is the other participant in an emotional experience which defines his identity in relation to the other and, as a result, impacts on the identification process of the other.

The killing of a woman, as a tragic outcome of a spiral of violence perpetrated by subjects close to the victim like her husband or ex-partner, clearly illustrates how some of the skills women reveal in the public sphere, like empathy and a willingness to donate are reshaped in their intimate lives, becoming veritable "corrosive disadvantages" of an emotional-affective type. The victim trusts and activates receptive mechanisms before and endurance afterwards, by virtue of the fact that the perpetrator is (or has been) almost always her partner. And this clearly makes perception of how violence, even before it erupts, is present at symbolic level of dominant, often shared representations. As Franca Bimbi writes "in late modernity and in the regime of equal opportunities it is necessary to keep in mind that symbolic violence lies between what we permit without realizing it and what we intimately dissent from without being able to express it" (Bimbi & Basaglia, 2010: 33).

Which leaves us to hypothesize how particular emotional attitudes can favour the acceptance of *gender violence*. These are attitudes that do not belong to the rational domain of reflective activity, but to a more visceral dimension determined by ancestral representations that many women struggle hard, but often fail to neutralize. They belong to a veritable symbolic device capable of shaping emotions by adapting them to an invisible and unconscious image of what it means to be a woman, but evident in its effects; a perceptual system located between premodern representations and late-modernizing pressures that makes practices which the victims would consider unacceptable in public life, plausible.

This induces us to reflect on the emotional sphere of women, more empathetic and morally constrained by male instrumental rationality, because this sphere is strongly conditioned by a system of reputation and social recognition which unites public life and the stability of private life, without reckoning with the decline of the male in the public sphere and the sometimes violent attempts of *recovery* of status they make in the private sphere to the detriment of their partners or ex-partners.

These are emotions of which women are bearers and which support abilities that can be neutralized or manipulated, precisely because they belong to the experience of all of us. These abilities make life truly human, but, at the same time, they are subject to everything else the other, as an acknowledged subject, plans and implements to encourage their development or, otherwise, to hinder their growth.

If on the one hand, the concept of ability is intended in its universalistic sense, on the other hand it is subordinated to specific situations that can facilitate or prevent its development.

Therefore, there are capacities, skills "that can prove useful when facilitating others" (Nussbaum, 2012: 138) as well as acting as disadvantages that may be added to others (corrosive disadvantages precisely). From this point of view, skills are a perishable and impractical asset when it comes to oppressive contexts because of being "irreducibly plural" disadvantages; all the more so, if we consider the emotional heritage available to us as one of the abilities indicated by Martha Nussbaum and, therefore, "as the intrinsic possibility for each person, to be able to establish links with people and things beyond and outside of ourselves; to be able to love those who love and care for us, to suffer because of their absence; in general, loving, suffering, feeling lacking, gratitude and justified anger" (ibidem) together with life, physical health, physical integrity, the senses, imagination and thought, practical reason, union with people and with living creatures, the ability to play and, at the same time, to take control of their environment (Nussbaum, 2004, 2007, 2010). It is something that is legitimized by a production of meaning that renders specific patterns of behaviour and attitudes recognizable within situations or "provinces of meaning" (Schütz, 1932). Such are the pre-eminent worlds of real objects and events in which we can take hold with our actions and, therefore, in the "mutual play of structures of relevance" (ibidem), through which an object or event becomes a theme or topic of our thinking. It is precisely the "provinces of meaning" which deem "adaptive preferences" *sui generis* because, unlike those posted by Marta Nussbaum, they do not promote "spheres of freedom" within the pluralism of different conceptions of life, but justify the *sui generis* workings of an oppressive–violent relationship.

Proximity violence highlights the corrosive disadvantages that arise when archaic and modern representations of the habitat impersonate overlap. It is intended as a constitutive, and therefore institutional, condition of the ego-alter relationship, capable of developing procedures aimed at recognizing the identity of each actor involved in the rituals that make a deviant situation acceptable. In an attempt to harmonize western and late-modern values with the cultural heritage of the Mediterranean that still make their influence felt in women's self-evaluation in relation to their own actability/ability to combine values deriving from Mediterranean models and post-modern values of self-autonomy, *gender violence* transforms abilities and skills into corrosive disadvantages, that is, into series of constitutive limitations that reduce human existence to perennial emotional failure.

The latter therefore *exercises institutional power within intimate relationships*, which thus become self-sufficient (1), autoimmune (2), and exclude conflict (3) in its manifold manifestations.

1. When violence – in its different forms and modes – becomes the very cement of the relationship, it assumes the characteristics of self-sufficiency. Violence, that is "sufficient" to keep the relationship up and running; within the behavioural ritual of the partners involved, it performs a constituent function allowing the relationship to continue. This is true both in the case of a couple's relationship and in relationships between teenagers or young people (where group-violence dynamics arise).
2. As an autoimmune phenomenon, a relationship based on violence excludes any other form of resistance to violence from within, as the latter becomes indispensable to maintaining the relationship. Thus, violence becomes the foundation upon which the domination of one over the other is based, when any other form of mutual and reciprocal attachment is lacking.
3. It replaces the conflict which – in its "domesticated" form of antagonism, competition, rivalry, and dialectic – provides for the "intentional symmetry" of the subjects involved in action aimed at obtaining a result or winning the stakes while, at the same time, it provides for "an asymmetry of objectives, expectations and resources used to find balance between the parties or a repositioning of the parts" (Bartholini, 2013: 18).

Insofar as it is self-sufficient, autoimmune and conflict-excluding, in the case of proximity violence unfavourable conditions of various kinds intersect and add and may be equated with the corrosive disadvantages identified by Nussbaum, which are, in our interpretation:

(a) *durée*, that is, a temporal continuity of the experiences regarding the interpersonal sphere of several subjects poised between pre-modern values and post-modern emancipatory drives;
(b) a state of *relational oppression* which may be considered as a possible identity-acknowledgement strategy constituting the context in which violence is reiterated and ritualized;
(c) *asymmetry of power* between a persecutor and the person persecuted which might be better defined as a form emotional blackmail based on the acknowledgement/contempt of identity proportional to how much a woman is capable of adapting to the symbolic violence of legacies of dominion in private life.[1]

When describing her approach to skills and ability, Martha Nussbaum focuses, above all, on concrete forms of safeguard that may translate into options of escape from situations of violence legitimized by intimate relationships and hampered by the corrosive disadvantages that may prevent this exit. If when an Indian woman

[1] For a broader and more detailed reflection on the categories of violence indicated above, see Bartholini (2019).

tells her story she describes how "during marriage Vasanti was cut off from any relationship except that strongly unequal one with her violent husband" (Nussbaum, 2012: 17), she also notes that "a woman who owns land it is less likely to be beaten because that might end the marriage and lead to the loss of a valuable asset. Other forms of safeguard against an abusive husband are work, education, movable property and savings" (ibidem).

In the case of Western women, during our appraisal of their experiences and while reflecting on the lives of Western-Mediterranean women, victims of violence, we have become increasingly aware of how the forms of safeguard that need to be activated against that very emotional abduction they themselves helped produce in a condition of relational oppression, are also and above all of an emotional-cultural type. In other words, this situation is the outcome of the clash between late-modern and neo-patriarchal cultures of which the women feel the impact and which forces them to adopt an amphibiotic habitus making them, the one hand, professional workers located adequately in the public sphere, partners emotionally subjected to male diktats in the private one.

Not only thanks to research carried out previously (Bartholini, 2013 and subsequent publications), but during participant observation conducted in recent years as a friend, colleague and fellow-researcher of many women, it was possible to note that the more women achieved their goals in the professional field, the more they allowed themselves to be ensnared by feelings of inferiority and inadequacy with respect to the habitus adopted in their partnerships. This conditioned their choices and behaviour up to the point of accepting their partners' prevaricating diktats the effects of which were clearly reflected in the emotional sphere.

6.6 Conclusions

Therefore, if one views the *violence suffered in the intimate dimension of proximity relationships* as a legacy inherited from patriarchal cultures now devoid of *raison d'etre*, one fails to enter in depth into one of the interpretative keys of the present "state of health" of intimate relationships, of public–private chiasma underlying it in a cultural area where Atlantic and Mediterranean paradigms intersect. Today, it is impossible to take the end of male hegemony for granted and consider the phenomenologies of men's violence against women in "our" world as pre-modern. Despite the increase in cases where women, besides holding important positions in the professional sphere, are themselves a family's *sole female breadwinner*, episodes and behaviour marked, indirectly, by gender violence are not infrequent. In these cases, violence is conveyed through discourse and images which, by radicalizing themselves, denote models of male domination (Bourdieu, 1998, 2015) within relations between men and women which converge only prima facie while, in reality, they are strongly asymmetrical with the female "giving" and voluntarily offering herself up to a dramaturgy of submission, in an attempt to gratify her partner and sanctioning her distance from certain premodern representations that still weigh on her imagination. Such images, although rationally circumscribed by awareness of being and feeling master of themselves, still weigh on the perceptual dimension with which many women, to use an expression of Nussbaum's, have "the strange feeling of having been robbed of a history, of no longer being people with a family history" (Nussbaum, 2016: 39–40), despite the fact that the cost of continuing a relational story may foresee the possibility of their own death at the hand of their partners, like the murder of "Sara", a student burnt alive by her ex-boyfriend. In rereading the statements of friends and family, Sara showed infinite compassion and rare pity for that young man from whom she had separated, compassion and pity that led her to bear with his threats, ambushes, stalking, and blackmail (Giomi & Magarragia, 2017).

Lorena was a very young student who in a few months would have graduated in medicine with a thesis in paediatrics. She was strangled by her boyfriend, a nurse: "I killed her because she gave me Coronavirus," he said to the investigators. Lorena had agreed to move to Furci, a small town in the provinces, for the love of her boyfriend who worked in that area after having got to know him in the corridors of the General Teaching Hospital in Messina. She worked in the wards where Covid19 patients were being treated. "Lorena was a passionate student. Her last message posted on Facebook three days earlier, spoke of the doctors who had been killed by Coronavirus. There she had launched an appeal: Now, more than ever before you need to show responsibility and love for life. Respect yourself, your families and your country" (La Repubblica 31/3/2020: 3).

Sara, a "brilliant" girl as her mother defined her (La Repubblica, 7/6/2015: 2), as well as by those who knew her, could sever the bond by expurgating from her inner life every emotion destined to translate into one "corrosive disadvantage", separating memories from the present? And could Lorraine accept being threatened and treated like a farmer instead of turning away from a man who accused her of "infecting" her like a witch of the Middle Ages or an accabadora who brings death?

Could Sara, defined as a "brilliant" girl by her mother (La Repubblica, 7/6/2015: 2) and by those who knew her, have severed the bond by purging from her intimate life every kind of emotion destined to translate into a "corrosive disadvantage" separating memories from the present? And could Lorraine have accepted being threatened and treated as an infector instead of turning away from the man who accused her of "infecting" him like some Mediaeval witch or *Accabadora* bringing death?

They both might have. However, neither Sarah nor Lorraine could not sever the links with their perpetrators in time, nor could all those victims of violence for whom the "intelligence of emotions" – oriented towards acknowledgement of others – became the warp of their own deadly trap.

In the same way, we tend to underestimate the deviant though substantial contribution violence itself, acting not only at concrete level, but also on an indirect and symbolic plane, to make sure the relationship "holds" (Bartholini, 2013).

From this angle, the Mediterranean area represents an intrinsic and peculiar field of analysis, "a geopolitical and geocultural space standing at a crucial crossroads, that of being either an area of perpetual disorder and destabilization or of transforming itself into a laboratory where new social relations may be experimented" (Pepicelli, 2007: 330). In it, the reality that arises in relation to the way men and women represent themselves and others within the context of their actions (Berger & Luckmann, 2000) and within their "provinces of meaning" (Schütz, 1932), is continually at the mercy of all those pre-modern legacies in conflict with the emancipatory process of women in the public sphere and which, acting upon their emotional sphere, makes them victims – even if only potential – of male violence, disarticulating their capability for autonomy and gender dignity.

What remain open are issues and problems referring to the social construction of violence, its incorporation into the "habitus" of men and women, the persistence of mechanisms of male domination expressed in the subjectivity of the victims or in their mental structures. These take the form, precisely, of categories of perception and emotional evaluation referring, nonetheless, to women from the European-Mediterranean area, their emancipation in the public and professional sphere. These are two *gender regimes* which attack "dignity as a reflective awareness of one's own uniqueness and moral autonomy [...] and the "honourable" space where European women are located" (Bimbi & Basaglia, 2010: 38–41).

Acknowledgement of the need to promote gender equality in the struggle against violence does not only mean fighting the multiple forms of disadvantage that half of the people find themselves suffering, in various forms and more or less marked ways, in different areas of the world and in ours. It means projecting oneself towards a model of society that imagines itself different precisely because of those gender skills which should not be translated into corrosive disadvantages of an emotional type for women who are bearers of an amphibiotic habitus. Such women, teetering between the western paradigm of emancipation and that of the Mediterranean tradition, are taught to become simultaneous generators of skills within the public sphere and bearers of those emotional disadvantages within the intimate-private one destined to demolish and destroy their selves in an effort to combine the intricate aspects of antithetical representations of womanhood in a Mediterranean and European area. Referring again to the "tightrope walker" painted by Chagall, we conclude by recalling that even in those paintings, things are not as they should be: the cocks are gigantic and the women walk upside down. In the emotional amphibiotics that only sleep should legitimize, fantasy overcomes the reality and the idealized memory of the past becomes more important than the present that is experienced with enorm*ous weariness.*

References

Balandier, G. (1994). *Le dédale. Pour en finir avec le XX siècle*. Paris, France: Fayard.

Balibar, E. (2001). Outlines of a topography of cruelty: Citizenship and civility in the era of global violence. *Constellations, 8*(1), 15–29.

Bartholini, I. (2013). *Violenza di prossimità. La vittima, il carnefice, lo spettatore e il "grande occhio"*. Milan, Italy: FrancoAngeli.

Bartholini, I. (2014). Gender violence in the Post-patriarchalization of global age: A comparative perspective of Italy and Serbia. *Zbornik Instituta za kriminološka i sociološka istraživanja, XXIII*(2), 25–38.

Bartholini, I. (2015). Introduzione a Id. (Ed.). *Violenza di genere e percorsi mediterranei. Voci, saperi, uscite*. Milan, Italy: Guerini e Associati.
Bartholini, I. (2016). Le parole della violenza. Recrudescenze mediterranee di patriarcalismo e sessismo. In F. Corbisiero (Ed.), *Genere e linguaggio. Le parole dell'uguaglianza e della diversità* (pp. 126–137). Milan, Italy: FrancoAngeli.
Bartholini, I. (2019). *Proximity violence in migration times. A focus in some regions of Italy, France, Spain*. Milano, Italy: FrancoAngeli.
Bauman, Z. (2000). *Liquid modernity*. Cambridge, UK: Polity Press.
Beck, U. (1998). *World risk society*. Cambridge, UK: Polity Press.
Berger, P. T., & Luckmann, T. (2000). *La realtà come costruzione sociale*. Bologna, Italy: Il Mulino (ed. orig. 1969).
Bimbi, F. (a cura di) (2003). Differenze e disuguaglianze. Prospettive per gli studi di genere in Italia. Bologna, Italy: Il Mulino.
Bimbi, F. (2015). *Onore e vergogna. Il ritorno di un paradigma mediterraneo nel dibattito europeo*. In I. Bartholini (a cura di), *Violenza di genere e percorsi mediterranei. Voci, saperi, uscite* (pp. 27–45). Milan, Italy: Guerini e Asssociti.
Bimbi, F., & Basaglia, A. (a cura di) (2010). Violenza contro le donne. Formazione di genere e migrazioni globalizzate. Milan, Italy: Guerini e Associati.
Bourdieu, P. (1979). *Le Sens pratique*. Paris, France: Minuit.
Bourdieu, P. (1998). *Masculine domination*. Stanford: University Press.
Bourdieu, P. (2015). *Il dominio maschile*. Milan, Italy: Feltrinelli (ed. orig. 1998).
Cassano, F., & Zolo, D. (Eds.). (2007). *L'alternativa mediterranea*. Milan, Italy: Feltrinelli.
Collins, R. (2014). *Violenza. Un'analisi sociologica*. Catanzaro, Italy: Rubettino (ed. orig. 2008).
Connel, R. W., & Messerschmidt, J. W. (2005). Hegemonic masculinity: Rethinking the concept. *Gender and Society, 19*(6), 829–859.
Corradi, C. (2009). *Sociologia della violenza. Modernità, identità, potere*. Rome, Italy: Meltemi.
Giddens, A. (1992). *The transformation of intimacy*. Cambridge, UK: Polity Press.
Giddens, A. (2000). *Runaway world*. London: Routledge.
Giomi, E., & Magarragia S. (2017). Relazioni Brutali. *Genere e violenza nella cultura mediale*. Bologna, Italy: Il Mulino.
Giordano, C. (2005). Mediterranean honor and beyond. The social management of reputation in the public sphere. *Sociologija Mintis ir Veiksmas, 1*, 40–55.
Gracia, E., & Lila, M. (2015). *Attitudes towards violence against women in EU*. Luxembourg, Luxembourg: Publication Office of the European Union.
Greverus, I. M., Romhild, R., & Welz, G. (2001). Reworking the past, shaping the present, considering the future. An introduction to the two issues of 'the Mediterraneans'. *Anthropological Journal on European Cultures, 10*, 1–10.
Habermas, J. (1985). *Il discorso filosofico della modernità*. Rome, Italy/Bari, Italy: Laterza (ed. orig. 1982).
Hanmer, J., & Itzin, C. (Eds.). (2001). *Trusht about domestic violence: Feminist influences on policy and practice*. New York: Routledge.
Honneth, A. (1995). *The struggle for recognition: The moral grammar of social conflicts*. Oxford, UK: Polity Press.
Inglehart, R. (2018). *Cultural evolution: People's motivations are changing, and reshaping the world*. Cambridge, UK: University Press.
Kimmel, M. S. (2000). *The gendered society*. Oxford, UK: University Press.
Monckton-Smith, J. (2012). Murder, gender and the media. In *Narratives of dangerous love*. London: Palgrave Macmillan UK.
Nussbaum, M. C. (2004). Emotions as judgments of value and importance. In R. C. Solomon (Ed.), *Thinking about feeling* (pp. 183–199). Oxford, UK: Oxford University Press.
Nussbaum, M. (2004). *Hiding from humanity disgust, shame, and the law*. Princeton: Princeton University Press. https://archive.org/details/hidingfromhumani00mart.

Nussbaum, M. C. (2007). Constitutions and capabilities. "Perception" against lofty formalism. *Harward Law Review, CXXI*, 4–97.
Nussbaum, M. C. (2010). *From disgust to humanity: Sexual orientation and constitutional law*. Oxford, UK/New York: Oxford University Press.
Nussbaum, M. (2012). *The new religious intolerance: overcoming the politics of fear in an anxious age*. Cambridge, Massachusetts: Belknap Press of Harvard University. https://archive.org/details/newreligious_nuss_2012_000_10710563.
Nussbaum, M. (2016). *Anger and Forgiveness: Resentment, Generosity, Justice*. New York, N.Y.: Oxford University Press.
Pepicelli, R. (2007). Donne e diritti nel Mediterraneo. In F. Cassano & D. Zolo (Eds.), *L'alternativa mediterranea* (pp. 315–333). Milan, Italy: Feltrinelli.
Peristiany, J. G. (Ed.). (1965). *Honor and shame: The values of Mediterranean society*. London: Weidenfeld & Nicolson.
Pinker, S. (2011). *The better angels of our nature: Why violence has declined*. Montreal, QC: Viking.
Reyneri, E. (2011). *Sociologia del mercato del lavoro*. Bologna, Italy: Il Mulino.
Saraceno, C., & Keck, W. (2011). Towards an integrated approach for the analysis of gender equity in policies supporting paid work and care responsibilities. *Demographic Research, 25*(11), 371–406.
Sassen, S. (1999). *Guests and aliens*. New York: New Press.
Schütz, A. (1932). *Der sinnhafte Aufbau der sozialen Welt. Eine Einleitung in die verstehende Soziologie*. Wien, Austria: Springer.
Thapar-Björkert, S. (2007). *State policy, strategies and implementation in combating patriarchal violence, focusing on "honour related" violence*. Norrköping, Sweden: Integrationsverket.
Walter, N. (2010). *Living dolls. The return of sexism*. London: Virago Press.
Wright, R. T., & Decker, S. (1997). *Armed robbers in action. Stickups and street culture*. Lebanon, NH: Northeastern University Press.

Conclusions: The Violence Trap

The perception of proximity violence links migrant women and European women who live in the peripheral areas of Mediterranean European cities by the slim thread of emotions (Connell, 2007). Warm perceptions and hot emotions, as we have endeavoured to highlight in this volume, are cultivated independently in "spheres of sociability" where vulnerability and resistance mingle. They are not simplistically favoured by the geographical position of the places where they are generated, but rather by the ways in which mechanisms of sex and gender impact upon relative social and cultural contexts.

There still remains a question to be resolved regarding proximity violence, extraneous to the cultural, social, and civil development of women, even where they show that they have pursued in full an emancipatory pathway making them capable professionals and people who fit perfectly into to a mature kind of society.

There is a borderline between emancipation and subordination that lies beyond the situational and contextual dynamics which can be identified through the eyes of the researcher. Migrant women, especially those born in countries of Sub-Saharan Africa, said that they feel themselves confined in "subaltern positions". The Mediterranean-European women of the *Ballarò* district declared that those relationships which consider migrant women subordinate because of their vulnerability are not so "indisputably execrable". They insinuated that maybe their own personal condition may be more fragile and exposed to the contingency of vulnerability than that of migrant women, protected by the shield of their conjugal union. Here the lens through which each one observes the other has revealed the deepest, most secret trap of the metamorphosis of that very same violence, preserved for centuries within the frame of proximal relationships. This is tantamount to considering stability of a relationship experienced thanks to proximity violence as an experience which permits women to feel strong in their vulnerability and resistant in their defence of the simulacrum of the identity of the couple to which they belong.

This volume has explored the way migrant women are addressing, resisting, and ultimately challenging the misfortune of an emancipation that goes hand in hand

I. Bartholini, *The Trap of Proximity Violence*,
https://doi.org/10.1007/978-3-030-52451-7

with the need for hot emotions. It identified a series of strategies related to the processes of resistance that the "other women", victims of violence, devise to minimize negative self-representations of themselves.

During the development of the research carried out, it was noticed how migrant women's practices and strategies of daily resistance can act as the basis of an act of social relegation undermining the emancipatory pathway of European-Mediterranean women and crystallizing the gender imbalances of migrant women.

The concept of proximity brings into play something more complex which is not limited to the category of gender, but to the intimate and retrospective ones of the imagination and of nostalgia as a retroactive emotion and inadequacy with respect to internalized images.

Proximity is a concept acting as a "bridge" between two identities, that of the victim and that of the perpetrator reflecting what is inherent in each of them and mirrored in the universe surrounding each of them. It regards a number of dimensions. Proximity violence is indicative of interpersonal tension, the power of which is symbolic and the actualization, which the context favours and structure, is material and physical. It indicates an interconnection between a dimension of political domination and a private space of the imagination that ends up justifying violence. It indicates, at the same time, a violence rooted in *Lebenswelt* and which acquires greater visibility precisely in the weakest interstices of everyday life, domestic or intimate and private. It denotes the outcome of the victim's recognition of the other within a context that justifies violence by virtue of the same institutional vulnerability that produces the necessary alibis. Finally, it feeds on trust and private abandonment that leads to abuse.

This volume has highlighted the deepest violence trap that is not in the relationship as such, but in the way we perceive that other who is our intimate enemy, a source of life even when it comes to a brutalized kind of life. The book highlights the difficulties encountered when observing the existence of each of us and attributing a different name to relationships precisely because each is lacerated by profound ambivalence: on the one hand we desire, we yearn for life as a couple, a life of love, on the other, we take refuge in surrogates of love which assume violence as a constitutive factor of a relationship, due to the difficulty of perceiving oneself as a subject without a relationship which permits one to mirror oneself in another.

The bitter and terrible truth of this age of ours is that perhaps that we women do not wish to abandon the irresistible tension that is created in a relationship of proximity violence, and that where it is wanting, one of the constitutive factors of being "present" due to the pathological attention of the other, necessary for the staging of the representation of love against the liquidity of love. Proximity violence makes each one necessary to the other; it is the fatigue, fear, and trembling existing within a relationship that is substantiated as "us". The trap is formed when we try to break the web of meaningless exhaustion and bitterness, which invades our lives daily and we fall as victims *ob torto collo* into a relationship of proximity violence fooling ourselves that this may make us visible, non-interchangeable, non-transient.

The protagonist of Erika Jong's novel, *Parachutes and Kisses* (1984), in her arduous struggle to gain independence, to become capable of having an *adult* relationship with her man, to her daughter, who, while listening to the tale of the *Sleeping Beauty*, asks her "What if the prince doesn't come?", replies that the sleeping beauty will have to wake up alone and hug herself tightly.

In becoming an instrument which others may use, there is perversion of false love and of a relationship that does not foresee the possibility of having a *You* with whom to communicate. One cannot do without resistance and approach the dark side of one's vulnerability except by opening the "sealed jar" of fear of one's own inadequacy. In violence, the victim is always sufficiently adequate to her own role, it suffices to undergo, resist, and remain. Avoiding a violent tie presumes dealing with the difficulty of relating to oneself, a vulnerability of a different kind, that of solitude which offers the possibility of knowing and accepting ourselves and, in the end, of loving ourselves authentically. It is much easier to be faithful to a truth as illusory as it is shared in a relationship. It is much easier to be able not to desire the harm of the other when one is in a relationship which positions one as victim, resistant victim, and vulnerable victim. When one is not in a relationship, one becomes nostalgic for the role which permitted one to hide one's own indignity from oneself, one's perverse traits, the possibility of behaving in the worst possible way outside of the magical circle of proximity violence.

Self-acceptance of one's vulnerability and recognition of the mechanisms of resistance is a slow and difficult process to implement but it is also the only one that can prevent nostalgia for the liturgies of sacrifice of those *ecclesias* that feed on the body (and soul) of women. This is perhaps the road that can lead to independence, permitting the possibility of a symmetrical and fair *relationship* on the level of gender closeness. This seems to be the only way to "save one's life" and leap beyond the violence trap.

Reference

Connell, R. (2007). *Southern theory: The global dynamics of knowledge in social science*. Sydney. A&U Academic.

Index

I. Bartholini, *The Trap of Proximity Violence*,
https://doi.org/10.1007/978-3-030-52451-7

The manufacturer's authorised representative in the EU is Springer Nature Customer Service Centre GmbH, Europaplatz 3, 69115 Heidelberg, Germany. If you have any concerns regarding our products, please contact ProductSafety@springernature.com

Printed and bound by CPI Group (UK) Ltd, Croydon, CR0 4YY
30/09/2026
02225709-0003